IMMUNOBIOLOGY AND PATHOGENESIS OF PERSISTENT VIRUS INFECTIONS

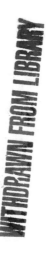

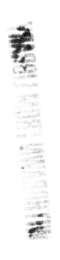

IMMUNOBIOLOGY AND PATHOGENESIS OF PERSISTENT VIRUS INFECTIONS

Edited by

Brian W. J. Mahy

Division of Viral and Rickettsial Diseases
Centers for Disease Control and Prevention
Atlanta, Georgia

and

Richard W. Compans

Department of Microbiology and Immunology
Emory University School of Medicine
Atlanta, Georgia

harwood academic publishers
Australia • Canada • China • France • Germany • India • Japan
Luxembourg • Malaysia • The Netherlands • Russia • Singapore
Switzerland • Thailand • United Kingdom

ABF8310

OCT 1 7 1997

Emmaplein 5
1075 AW Amsterdam
The Netherlands

British Library Cataloguing in Publication Data

Immunobiology and pathogenesis of persistent virus
    infections
    1. Immunology 2. Immune system 3. Medical virology 4. Virus
    diseases – Immunological aspects
    I. Mahy, B. W. J. (Brian Wilfred John) II. Compans, Richard
    W.
    616'.079

    ISBN   3–7186–0607–0 (hardcover)
           3–7186–0622–4 (softcover)

CONTENTS

INTRODUCTION

Viruses from diverse families, which exhibit marked differences in their structural properties and replication processes, may have the common feature of causing long-term persistent infection in man and other natural hosts. With some viruses, a long-term persistent infection is the normal outcome of infection, and the progression of the disease process may occur over many years. Other viruses usually cause acute, self-limiting infection with only occasional establishment of long-term persistence. With many viruses that can cause persistent infection, the host immune response may be an important component in inducing tissue damage. The mechanisms involved in establishment and maintenance of persistent viral infections, and the interaction of such viruses with the immune system, are the focus of this volume. Five distinct groups of viruses — each of which is involved in the etiology of important human diseases — are discussed.

The lentiviruses subfamily of retroviruses shares several common properties, including a relatively long period between the acute stages of infection and the progression of clinical disease. Some viruses, such as HIV, cause immune deficiency, whereas others produce lymphoproliferative diseases or anemia. The mechanisms by which HIV infection can lead to depletion of CD4$^+$ T cells are discussed by J. Steven McDougal. This issue is fundamental to understanding the pathogenesis of AIDS and the susceptibility to opportunistic infections. It will be of great importance to dissect the relative significance of the alternative mechanisms of T cell depletion, which are dealt with in this chapter. Janice E. Clements et al. describe their studies on gene expression of another lentivirus, visna virus, which causes a progressive neurological disease of sheep. The role of macrophage infection and cytokine responses in the induction of disease in specific target organs is reported. William A. Blattner provides an overview of the epidemiology of human retroviruses, contrasting the epidemiology and diseases induced by HTLV-I and II with that of HIV. The HTLV's are excellent systems through which to study viruses that persist for extremely long periods before disease induction.

Varicella zoster virus (VZV) establishes latency in cells of the dorsal root ganglia following primary virus infection. Reactivation of the virus results in herpes zoster, involving extensive inflammatory responses and cytopathology in the dorsal ganglia cells. Ann M. Arvin explains her recent studies on identifying major VZV proteins that are recognized by human T cells. Long-lived CTL responses are induced by infection as well as by experimental vaccines.

Measles virus usually causes an acute, self-limited infection; however, persistent infection can occur in some instances. Studies of measles virus pathogenesis carried out in two laboratories, including analysis of gene expression and virus-immune cell interactions, are reviewed by Sibylle Schneider-Schaulies et al. Several possible mechanisms by which measles virus may induce autoimmune responses and their possible role in pathogenesis are discussed. Diane E. Griffin et al. describe the interaction of measles virus with the immune system. Results indicate that after acute infection, measles virus preferentially induces a type 2 CD4$^+$ T cell response, resulting in high levels of antibody responses, and low levels of CTL responses. Measles has remained a persistent problem in human populations worldwide, especially in underdeveloped countries; vaccine coverage there is poor, and more than a million deaths result from measles every year. The reemergence in 1989 of large numbers of measles cases and a significant number of deaths in the United States prompted new control measures; and since 1991 a second dose of measles vaccine has been given to school-age children in addition to universal infant vaccination at 15 months of age. William Bellini and his group have used gene sequencing to analyze the impact of this control strategy on the circulation of measles in the U.S. population. They conclude that indigenous measles transmission has effectively ceased, whereas measles outbreaks continue to occur as a result of measles virus importations from other countries.

Hepatitis B virus often causes persistent infection, which may lead to hepatic cell carcinoma. William S. Robinson reviews mechanisms of

HBV persistence and disease induction, including potentially oncogenic genetic changes found in different species or associated with different hepatitis B viruses. Some of these represent direct viral effects, whereas others appear not to be caused by a direct viral mechanism. The interaction of HBV with hepatic cells is described by Wolfram H. Gerlich and Xuanyong Lu, with particular emphasis on virus attachment and possible mechanisms of virus penetration.

Unlike the viruses discussed above, where man is the primary host, many other viruses infect humans and cause diseases without significant inter-human spread. One such group of vector-borne viruses includes the agents that cause hemorrhagic fever. C. J. Peters and James W. LeDuc report on the mechanisms involved in persistence in animal reservoirs of Rift Valley fever virus, hantaviruses, and arenaviruses, all of which are RNA viruses involved in the etiology of hemorrhagic fevers. Lisa Lau and Rafi Ahmed review recent studies on antiviral CD8[+] cytotoxic T cell memory in mice infected with lymphocytic choriomeningitis virus, another arenavirus. They present the important finding that cytotoxic T cell memory does not require persistent antigenic stimulation, but rather requires the generation of long-lived antigen-independent memory T cells. These results are also relevant to the development of novel immunization strategies.

A better understanding of the mechanisms of viral persistence is essential for developing new approaches to control viral diseases, including novel approaches for vaccine development. The contributors to this book sincerely hope that it will point the way to future directions in research toward these important objectives.

CONTRIBUTORS

Rafi Ahmed, University of California School of Medicine, Los Angeles

Ann M. Arvin, Stanford University School of Medicine, Stanford, California

William J. Bellini, Centers for Disease Control and Prevention, Atlanta, Georgia

Martin A. Billeter, Institute for Molecular Biology, Zürich, Switzerland

William A. Blattner, Institute of Human Virology, Baltimore, Maryland

Lucy M. Carruth, Johns Hopkins University School of Medicine, Baltimore, Maryland

Janice E. Clements, Johns Hopkins University School of Medicine

Lisa M. Esolen, Johns Hopkins University School of Medicine

Susan L. Gdovin, University of Maryland, College Park

Wolfram H. Gerlich, University of Giessen, Germany

Diane E. Griffin, Johns Hopkins University School of Medicine

Lisa L. Lau, University of California School of Medicine, Los Angeles

James W. LeDuc, World Health Organization, Geneva, Switzerland

Xuanyong Lu, University of Giessen

J. Steven McDougal, Centers for Disease Control and Prevention

C. J. Peters, Centers for Disease Control and Prevention

William S. Robinson, Stanford University School of Medicine

Jürgen Schneider-Schaulies, University of Würzburg, Germany

Sibylle Schneider-Schaulies, University of Würzburg

Jens-Jörg Schnorr, University of Würzburg

Volker ter Meulen, University of Würzburg

Brian J. Ward, Johns Hopkins University School of Medicine

1

Mechanisms of CD4 T cell depletion in human immunodeficiency virus type 1 infection

J. Steven McDougal

Immunology Branch, Division of HIV/AIDS, National Center for Infectious Disease, Centers for Disease Control and Prevention, U.S. Department of Health and Human Services, Public Health Service, Atlanta, GA 30333, USA

Introduction

Since the earliest reports of the acquired immunodeficiency syndrome (AIDS), it has been appreciated that the central immune defect in this disease is a numerical/functional loss of T cells that express the cell surface marker, CD4. CD4 T cells perform critical recognition and induction functions in the immune response to foreign stimuli. Human immunodeficiency virus type 1 (HIV–1) infection results in gradual CD4 T cell depletion, progressive immune unresponsiveness with effective paralysis in virtually all arms of the immune system, and increasing susceptibility to opportunistic infections and malignancies. Thus, HIV–1 immunodeficiency is viewed from the immunologic perspective as a graded severity of CD4 T cell depletion, distributed on a continuum of time, influenced by incompletely understood cofactors, and associated with a spectrum of increasing clinical severity that reflects the severity of CD4 T cell depletion.

1

As with all persistent virus infections, there is a complex and dynamic interplay between the virus and the host response to infection. Clarification of how virus infection results in CD4 T cell depletion in the host is central to an understanding of the pathogenesis of this disease. In this review, fundamental characteristics of CD4 T cell function, the biology of HIV–1, the natural history of infection, and the problem of CD4 T cell depletion are summarized. These are followed by an itemization of factors that may account for or contribute to CD4 T cell depletion (Table 1). In particular, features of the host immune response are examined. Many immunologic features of this infection remain an enigma. Ten years after discovery of the virus, it is still not always possible to make a fundamental distinction between those features of the immune response that contribute to progressive disease and those features that limit or restrain progression in this seemingly inexorable disease.

Background: immunology and CD4 T cell function

The function of the immune system is to discriminate self from nonself. As a consequence of nonself recognition, cellular and humoral interactions are set in motion that result in the sequestration and elimination of that which is recognized as foreign or antigenic. The immune system is derived from two cell lineages: monocytic and lymphocytic. Monocytes and their tissue counterparts, macrophages, seed structures of the mononuclear phagocytic system (Kupffer cells, sinisoidal cells in the spleen, Langerhans cells in the skin, microglial cells in the brain, dendritic cells in lymph node and thymus, and the like). These cells have no innate antigen specificity but do scavenge antigens (especially particulate antigens) and present them in an immunogenic form to lymphoid cells. By virtue of receptors for immunoglobulin, complement, or lymphokines, monocyte-derived cells respond to mediators of the immune response and are recruited to mount an inflammatory attack on foreign antigens.

Lymphocytes are divided into two major cell types: T cells and B cells. B cells synthesize immunoglobulin and express it on their cell surface as integral membrane immunoglobulin. B cells are precursors of plasma cells, cells that secrete immunoglobulin. Mature T cells circulate from blood to tissue to lymph. They are relatively long-lived, and their recir-

Table 1.1. *Mechanisms of CD4 T cell depletion and functional impairment in HIV infection*

1. Death of individually infected cells

    a. Requires cell activation/viral replication

    b. The accumulation of intracellular CD4:gp120 complexes is toxic

2. Fusion of uninfected CD4 cells with HIV-infected cells

    a. Syncytia (fusion) formation

    b. Super-transmission by dendritic/monocytic cells

3. Immune recognition and reaction with HIV–1 and with HIV–1 infected cells

    a. Cytolytic T cell recognition (MHC-restricted CTL)

    b. Antibody-dependent cellular cytotoxicity (ADCC)

    c. C'-mediated cytolysis

    d. Antibody enhancement

4. Immune recognition of uninfected cells bearing viral products

    a. CTL recognition of CD4 cells that have processed soluble gp120

    b. ADCC of CD4 cells with absorbed gp120

5. Immunosuppression/depletion by viral products

    a. Perversion of specific CD4 T cell antigen recognition by gp120 absorbed to CD4: induction of programmed cell death (apoptosis)

6. Autoimmunity or aberrant immune reactivity

    a. Cross reacting viral/cellular antigens (gp120/MHC)

    b. Non-MHC-restricted cytolysis of activated CD4–T cells

    c. Anti-CD4 antibodies

    d. Idiotype-anti-idiotype interactions

    e. Superantigen

culation pattern is ideally suited for immune surveillance. Two T cell markers, CD2 and CD3, are found on most mature T cells and are referred to as pan-T cell markers. T cells can be further subdivided by two other phenotypic markers, CD4 and CD8, which are on mutually exclusive populations of T cells in the peripheral blood. Historically, CD4 and CD8 T cell populations have been associated with helper/inducer and cyto-toxic/suppressor functions, respectively. This remains a predominant association, although it is by no means absolute. A more stringent association of CD4 and CD8 phenotype with function is in the way they recognize antigen rather than in their subsequent effector functions. CD4 T cells recognize antigen that is processed and presented in the context of class II structures of the major histocompatibility complex (MHC). CD8 cells recognize antigen in the context of class I MHC structures. During T cell ontogeny in the thymus, double CD4/CD8-positive cells exist. These undergo a series of differentiation and selection steps, in which self-reac-tive cells are either eliminated or paralyzed (negative selection or toler-ance induction) or the cells acquire immunocompetence and emerge with cell-surface markers characteristic of mature T cells.

CD4 T cells are a pivotal cell in the orchestration of an effective im-mune response. They mount the initial specific immune response to anti-gen (processed and presented by antigen-presenting cells) and, in turn, induce other cells to perform their respective immunologic functions. They induce, prime or activate CD8 T cytotoxic cells, B cells, and mono-cyte-derived cells.

The T cell receptor (TCR) for antigen recognizes antigen presented in the context of MHC molecules, specifically antigen that is processed and presented within a groove in the MHC molecule (Figure 1). The TCR is coupled to the CD3 complex of proteins that transduce activation signals to the interior of the cell. As mentioned, CD4 T cells are strictly confined to class II MHC-restricted responses, a commitment established during thymic development. This process requires active selection, in which the CD4 molecule plays an essential role. The role of CD4 in antigen recog-nition by peripheral CD4 T cells is one of augmentation or amplification. CD4 has weak affinity for class II MHC and amplifies the interaction bet-ween T cells and antigen presenting cells. Coclustering of the TCR/CD3 complex amplifies responses, whereas separate crosslinking of CD4 and

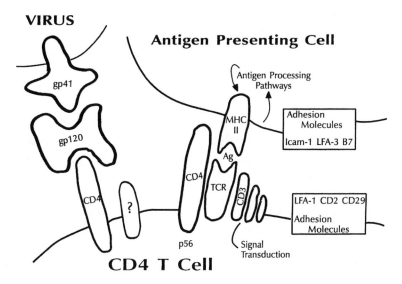

Figure 1.1 Schematic representation of CD4 T cell recognition of antigen (on the right) and the attachment of HIV–1 (on the left).

the TCR/CD3 complex may be a signal that induces tolerance. Both CD4 and CD8 are associated on their cytoplasmic tails with the protein tyrosine kinase, p56–lck. The zeta chain of the CD3 complex is one substrate of the p56 tyrosine kinase, providing a biochemical link between CD4 and TCR/CD3 activation.

Background: HIV–1 biology

Shortly after the discovery of the AIDS virus, HIV–1, it was appreciated that HIV–1 has a restricted tropism for CD4 cells and CD4+ cell lines *in vitro*. In addition to T cells, human monocytes express CD4 and can be infected with HIV (Nicholson et al., 1986; Koenig et al., 1986; Gartner et al., 1986). There is no restriction in the innate capacity of mammalian cells to replicate virus. Virtually all mammalian cells that have been tested will replicate infectious HIV–1 provided HIV is introduced into the cells as cloned and integrated proviral DNA by transfection (Levy, 1993; Cann et al., 1990; Levy et al., 1986; Fisher et al., 1985). The amount of viral replication but not the potential for replication does vary between cell types, presumably reflecting differences in the activation state of the cell and the induction of viral/host cell transcription factors. Therefore, the apparent preferential tropism of HIV for certain cell types must relate to events that occur before replication (attachment, penetration, reverse transcription or integration).

The basis for this restricted tropism lies in the necessity for a specific virus cell receptor interaction, namely the interaction of HIV–1 outer envelope protein gp120 with the CD4 molecule. Evidence that CD4 functions as a receptor for HIV–1 comes from several lines of investigation. Monoclonal antibodies to CD4 prevent infection of CD4 cells by HIV–1 (McDougal et al., 1985; Dalgleish et al., 1984; Klatzmann et al., 1984). Virus binds specifically to CD4 cells, and this binding is inhibited by anti-CD4 or anti-gp120 antibodies (McDougal et al., 1986b; McDougal et al., 1985). Bimolecular complexes of CD4 and gp120 are isolated from HIV–1-exposed CD4 T cells (McDougal et al., 1986a). Human cells that do not express CD4 and cannot be infected by HIV–1 are rendered susceptible by transfection and expression of CD4 cDNA (Maddon et al., 1986). Finally, soluble forms of the CD4 molecule block HIV binding and infectivity (Deen et al., 1988; Traunecker et al., 1988; Smith et al., 1987; Fisher et al., 1988; Hussey et al., 1988).

Although CD4 expression is necessary and sufficient for infection of human cell lines, there is a curious exception in rodent cell lines. Mouse cell lines expressing human CD4 cannot be infected with HIV–1 (Maddon et al., 1986). Experiments with mouse–human somatic cell hybrids indicate that a second (other than human CD4) human factor is required for infection (Broder et al., 1993; Dragic et al., 1992). The second receptor, more appropriately called a coreceptor, has not been identified. Facilitated entry has been reported wherein antibody-coated virions enter cells, especially macrophages, through their Fc– or complement receptors (Jiang et al., 1991; Boyer et al., 1991; Homsy et al., 1989; Takeda et al., 1988; Robinson et al., 1988; Montefiori et al., 1990; McKeating et al., 1990). Human macrophages express CD4, and it appears that so-called antibody enhancement of viral entry is not independent of CD4 (Connor et al., 1991; Perno et al., 1990; Takeda et al., 1990; Joualt et al., 1989) although it may be independent of CD4 in other cell types (Boyer et al.,

1991; Homsy et al., 1989; McKeating et al., 1990). Infectivity for some CD4–negative cell lines has also been reported and alternative receptors have been proposed (Joling et al., 1993; Qureshi et al., 1990; Harouse et al., 1991; Li et al., 1990; Cheng-Mayer et al., 1987; Homsy et al., 1989). Nevertheless, in vitro infection has been most reliably, efficiently, and reproducibly obtained only in CD4+ cells.

Binding of gp120 to CD4 is sufficient for viral infection, at least in human cells, although there may be other components that amplify the binding or promote the subsequent entry of virus (Figure 1). HIV–1 enters cells by fusion of viral and host cell membrane. For the most part, the mechanism of fusion resides in viral components and not in the CD4 component (Perez et al., 1992; Dubay et al., 1992; Helseth et al., 1990; Marsh and Dalgleish, 1987; Stein et al., 1987; Maddon et al., 1988; Gallaher, 1987; Kowalski et al., 1987; Sodroski et al., 1986). CD4 probably functions simply as a focusing agent for virus, overcoming repulsive forces between membranes and allowing fusion to take place. Additional secondary functions in entry have been ascribed to CD4 by some (Truneh et al., 1991; Celada et al., 1990; Moore et al., 1992; Poulin et al., 1991). CD4 is known to be involved in signal transduction pathways in the activation of T cells (vide supra). However, there is no evidence that CD4-mediated activation signals are required for the actual penetration event (Orloff et al., 1991b; Horak et al., 1990). An early report concluding that HIV–1 only infects activated cells and cannot infect resting, non-activated CD4 T cells (Gowda et al., 1989) is explained not by a block in entry but by a requirement for cellular activation after entry for complete reverse transcription of viral RNA into DNA (Orloff et al., 1991b; Zack et al., 1990).

Background: natural history and the problem of CD4 T cell depletion

A central question of pathogenesis is how HIV–1 infection results in massive CD4 T cell depletion in the host. An intuitive and perhaps simplistic (though personally favored) notion is that HIV infects and destroys CD4 T cells and that this accounts for the depletion. However, early studies indicate that too few cells harbor virus at any one time to account for the relatively large loss of CD4 cells (Harper et al., 1986). Later studies using

Natural History of HIV-1 Infection

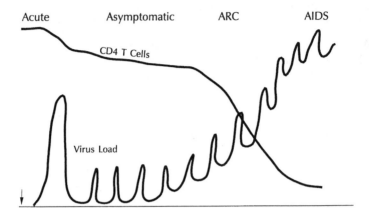

Figure 1.2   Natural history of HIV-1 infection. CD4 T cells decline and virus burden increases as the disease progresses.

more sensitive HIV DNA detection techniques indicate a larger proportion of cells may harbor virus making this a less compelling argument (Connor et al., 1993; Schnittman et al., 1990a; de Wolf et al., 1988; Bagasra et al., 1992). Nevertheless, a number of mechanisms that invoke more elaborate indirect mechanisms have been postulated, have been demonstrated in vitro, and are in accordance with physiologically relevant aspects of CD4 T cell function in the immune system.

Any explanation of the pathogenesis of HIV-1 infection has to account for two essential features that are associated with the natural history of this disease. First, CD4 T cells decline in association with more severe immunodeficiency and clinical progression. Secondly, it is now quite clear that progressive disease is associated with increasing viral load in patients (Connor et al., 1993; Schnittman et al., 1989; Schnittman et al., 1990a; de Wolf et al., 1988) (Figure 2). Progressive disease can also be associated with changes in the biologic properties and genetic diversity of the virus and with attendant changes in the immune responsiveness of the host.

Shortly after infection, there is a burst of virus replication and viremia (Graziosi et al., 1993; Daar et al., 1991; Clark et al., 1991; Roos et al., 1992). This is presumably responsible for dissemination of virus to lymphoid organs, brain, and other potential reservoirs of infection (i.e. virtually any organ containing monocyte-derived cells). Within weeks to months, a detectable immune response occurs associated with a decline in viremia. The patient then enters a period of relatively asymptomatic, clinical latency associated with slowly declining CD4 T cell levels and absent or episodic viremia. The duration of this state is variable and its determinants are not fully understood. However, it is not a state of true microbiologic latency (i.e. the presence of proviral DNA with no evidence for transcription). Though difficult to detect in peripheral blood, some level of viral replication persists throughout the course of infection, especially in lymphoid organs (Panteleo et al., 1993; Embretson et al., 1993; Armstrong and Horne, 1984; Panteleo et al., 1991). Clinical complications of AIDS are associated with a period of rapidly declining CD4 T cell levels, increasing viral burden (Connor et al., 1993; Schnittman et al., 1990a; de Wolf et al., 1988), a broadening of the genetic diversity of the virus (Holmes et al. 1992; Kuiken et al., 1992; Hahn et al., 1986; Saag et al., 1988; Willey et al., 1986), changes in the biologic properties of the virus (Groenink et al., 1991; Schuitemaker et al., 1992; Koot et al., 1993) and escape from immune attack (Treinblay and Wainberg, 1990; Albert et al., 1990; Arendrup et al., 1992; Phillips et al., 1991).

Mechanisms of CD4 T cell depletion

Death of individually infected cells

In vitro, infection of normal lymphocytes results in relatively rapid loss of CD4 T cells, a process that is hastened if the T cells are activated (McDougal et al., 1985; Folks et al., 1989; Tong-Starksen et al., 1989; Folks et al., 1986a; Folks et al., 1986b; Zagury et al., 1986; Cohen et al., 1992). If a CD4 cell is sufficiently activated in vitro such that substantial viral replication will ensue, the cell does not survive the insult. Lesser degrees of viral replication are compatible with symbiotic coexistence, particularly in some CD4 cell lines. Based on genetic manipulation of

virus and its introduction into various cell types, the minimum and sufficient requirements for cytopathicity are *env* gene expression by the virus
and CD4 expression by the infected cell (Kowalski et al., 1987; Lifson
et al., 1986a; Sodroski et al., 1986; Koga et al., 1990). Introduction of
HIV–1 into CD4-negative cells by transfection results in equivalent viral replication but no cell death (DeRossi et al., 1986). Similarly, certain
env mutants that cannot bind CD4 will replicate if introduced into CD4
cells, but cell death does not ensue (Thali et al., 1991). Using *env* gene
and CD4 gene constructs under the control of inducible promotors,
Koga et al. (1990) demonstrated that simultaneous expression of *env*
and CD4 was required and that the rapidity of cell death was a function
of the level of coexpression of the two. Thus the CD4:envelope interaction appears to be a requisite for cell death as well as for cell entry. Prior
to cell death, CD4 cells lose cell surface expression of CD4 (McDougal
et al., 1985; Hoxie et al., 1986). Intracellular complexes of CD4 and
gp120 accumulate when the infected cells have lost cell–surface expression of CD4 (Hoxie et al., 1986; Crise and Rose, 1992). Koga et al.
(1990, 1991) demonstrated that these complexes accumulated at the nuclear pores and suggest that interference with nuclear transport by the
complexes is responsible for cell death. The *vpu* gene product of HIV–1
is involved in dissociating intracellular gp120:CD4 complexes and de-
grading CD4 (Willey et al., 1992). This may be a mechanism that the
virus uses to partially subvert complex formation and cell death and allow for sufficient availability of gp120 for virus assembly. Similarly, the
nef gene product appears to down–regulate CD4 gene transcription
(Garcia and Miller, 1991; Guy et al., 1987).

Clearly, virus infection of a cell in the absence of extraneous extracellular factors (including the immune response to virus) is sufficient to
cause cell death provided intracellular conditions (activation) for ample
virus replication exist and the cell expresses the CD4 molecule. Whether
this is the sole explanation for CD4 T cell depletion in vivo may never be
answered. Nevertheless, the direct cell death theory is consistent with in
vivo observations (particularly the relationship between declining CD4 T
cell levels and increasing virus burden); it certainly could account for
CD4 T cell depletion on its own and must be considered a primary component of the disease process. From a practical standpoint, this mecha-

nism of pathogenesis supports a conventional therapeutic approach and is appealing because of its simplicity. Interventions should be aimed at reducing virus replication/spread and reducing inadvertent or unnecessary activation of susceptible cells. One need not invoke more elaborate extraneous factors or be sidetracked by possible epiphenomena that may require much more complicated strategies.

Sequestration of uninfected CD4 cells by HIV-infected cells

Mechanisms of CD4 T cell depletion that do not require productive infection by the doomed CD4 T cell have also been proposed. Infected cells fuse and form syncytia with uninfected CD4 cells, a phenomena equivalent to functional, if not actual, cell death. *Env* gene expression is required of the infected cell, and CD4 expression is required of its fusion partner (Lifson et al., 1986a; Sodroski et al., 1986; Lifson et al., 1986b). Dendritic cells, specialized antigen-presenting cells that reside in lymph nodes, are particularly potent sources of HIV transmission to CD4 T cells (Cameron et al., 1992). It has been argued that a mechanism by which infected cells sequester uninfected cells may explain how massive CD4 T cell depletion can occur when so few cells with demonstrable HIV–1 are detected in vivo. Furthermore, the efficiency of syncytium formation by virus strains bears a relationship to disease progression (Schuitemaker et al., 1992; Koot et al., 1993).

Structures consistent with HIV–1-containing syncytia have been observed in vivo, but they are certainly not a frequently observed feature of the disease's histopathology (Armstrong and Horne, 1984) except in brain (Sharer et al., 1985). However, the relative importance of syncytia formation versus direct viral destruction of individually infected cells in explaining CD4 T cell depletion remains to be determined.

Immune recognition and reaction with HIV–1 and with HIV–1-infected cells

The immune recognition and elimination of infected cells or cell-free virus would generally be viewed as beneficial, and this is probably the case in HIV infection. However, there is precedence for the immune response to a virus, rather than the virus per se, to be the cause of the pathology. Hepatitis B virus infection is a case in point. HIV-infected cells can be targets for cytolytic T cells. Both CD8, MHC class I restricted, and CD4, MHC class II restricted cytolytic T cells can be detected in HIV–1 infected people (Takahashi et al., 1989; Orentas et al., 1990; Johnson et al., 1992; Walker et al., 1987; Takahashi et al., 1988; Nixon et al., 1988; Polydefkis et al., 1990; Plata et al., 1987). Infected cells bearing viral proteins bind anti-HIV antibodies and thus become targets for cells that mediate antibody-dependent cellular cytotoxicity (ADCC) (Weinhold et al., 1989; Ljunggren et al., 1987; Ruscetti et al., 1986; Weinhold et al., 1988). Infected cells are not lysed efficiently by the addition of antibody and complement although complement-mediated lysis has been demonstrated (Spear et al., 1993; Gregersen et al., 1990; Spear et al., 1990).

Antibody enhancement of HIV–1 infectivity, with or without complement fixation, has been described (Jiang et al., 1991; Boyer et al., 1991; Homsy et al., 1989; Takeda et al., 1988; Robinson et al., 1988; Montefiori et al., 1990; McKeating et al., 1990). Although antibody-reactive epitopes of HIV–1 that are neutralizing and dominant epitopes that are non-neutralizing have been described, epitopes that consistently induce enhancing antibodies have not been identified (Levy, 1993). Antibody specificity appears to be less important than stoichiometry. In vitro, careful checkerboard titrations of HIV–1 and antibody are required to demonstrate the effect. In an in vivo environment of antibody excess, it seems unlikely that the prevailing effect would be enhanced infection. As mentioned, antibody-enhanced entry is not independent of CD4 in most cases (Connor et al., 1991; Perno et al., 1990; Takeda et al., 1990; Joualt et al., 1989). It seems likely that this in vitro phenomenon represents facilitated entry in which some concentrations of antibody, complement or both augment attachment to cell membranes for normal, CD4-mediated fusion. Independent uptake by Fc or C receptor pathways involves invagination of the receptor complex into phagosomes and subsequent phagosome–lysosome fusion, an environment that is likely to inactivate HIV–1 rather than promote its replication.

Is the HIV–1-specific immune response, intuitively viewed as beneficial, actually deleterious? There is little or no evidence that this paradox actually applies to HIV infection. Superficially, if HIV-specific immunity caused pathology, it should bear a relationship to disease progression. If anything, the opposite relationship is observed. In clinical studies, there appears to be a relationship between heightened immunity and long-term survival (Levy, 1993; Mackewicz et al., 1991; Homsy et al., 1990; Gotch et al., 1992) and, conversely, a relationship between deteriorating immunity to HIV and progressive disease (Levy, 1993; Mackewicz et al., 1991; McDougal et al., 1987; Nicholson et al., 1987; Fauci, 1993).

There is one possibility, perhaps little more than a curiosity, in which unique features of this virus and the immune response to it might result in the elimination of HIV-specific cells in a relatively selective way. Theoretically, HIV-specific CD4+ class II MHC-restricted T cell precursors would be induced in this disease. These cells would recognize activated (class II MHC-bearing) HIV-infected cells. Indeed, there could very well be a compounding effect on the affinity of interaction by virtue of two types of adhesion sites: TCR recognition of processed HIV antigen and the interaction of CD4 with envelope protein expressed by the infected cell (Figure 3). The potential for dual-site attachment may confer a selective recruitment of HIV-specific cells to HIV-infected targets. At the very least, a more avid interaction would occur between infected cells and HIV-specific CD4 T cells than between infected cells and CD4 T cells having other specificities. If the interaction results in fusion or infection of the responding cell (regardless of whether the target was destroyed in the process), preferential or selective elimination of HIV-specific CD4 cells may be the consequence. There is relatively little direct evidence for a preferential infectivity of HIV-specific CD4 cells in vivo. There is some evidence for infectivity of cells bearing certain beta-chain families of the TCR (Laurence et al., 1992) or for the preferential infection/depletion of certain functional subsets of CD4 cells (van Noesel et al., 1990; Schnittman et al., 1990b; Nicholson et al., 1984). It is, however, curious and consistent that HIV-specific, MHC restricted CD4 T cells are isolated more reliably from uninfected donors rather than from HIV-infected people, suggesting that perhaps there is a selective loss of HIV-specific CD4 cells in HIV infection (Orentas et al., 1990; Siliciano et al., 1988).

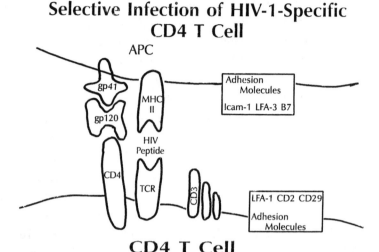

Selective Infection of HIV-1-Specific CD4 T Cell

Figure 1.3   Model for hypothetical selective infection of HIV-specific CD4 T cells by virus-infected antigen-presenting cells (APC). Dual site attachment occurs through TCR recognition of processed HIV antigen and the interaction of CD4 with gp120 expressed by the infected cell (see text).

Immune recognition of viral products that have been taken up by uninfected cells

The outer envelope protein, gp120, is noncovalently associated with the transmembrane protein, gp41. Gp120 is readily shed from HIV–1 and from HIV–1 infected cells and can adsorb to CD4 on uninfected cells. Uninfected CD4 T cells can take up and process gp120 for presentation to and recognition by cytolytic T cells (Siliciano et al., 1989; Lanzavecchia et al., 1988). Similarly CD4 cells can bind soluble gp120 and serve as targets, in vitro at least, for ADCC reactions (Weinhold et al., 1989; Weinhold et al., 1988). One need not wrestle with the theoretic problem posed in the previous section: is the immune attack on virus-infected cell beneficial because it stops further propagation or is it an important mechanism for depleting CD4 cells? In this mechanism, the CD4 cells are innocent bystanders; they are not productively infected. The problem here is to determine whether these reactions occur to any great extent in vivo. The levels of detectable soluble gp120 found in plasma are very low and certainly subsaturating. Similarly, it has not been possible to detect large amounts of cell surface gp120 on CD4 cells from infected patients using fluorescence detection methods. However, even very low levels of adsorbed gp120 may be sufficient to render a CD4 cell a target for cytolytic T cells or for cells mediating ADCC (Siliciano et al., 1989; Weinhold et al., 1989; Lanzavecchia et al., 1988).

Immunosuppression and induction of cell depletion by viral products

As mentioned, the CD4 molecule functions in the normal immune response by associating with the TCR/CD3 complex that recognizes antigen in association with class II MHC. Separate or prior cross-linking of CD4 by gp120 before antigen recognition and triggering by the TCR complex can depress responsiveness as measured by signal transduction events (Cefai et al., 1990; Mittler and Hoffmann, 1989; Linette et al., 1988; Hofmann et al., 1990; Orloff et al., 1991a), proliferation (Chirmule et al., 1990; Diamond et al., 1988; Pahwa et al., 1985; Wahl et al., 1989), and cytokine production (Oyaizu et al., 1990; Wahl et al., 1989) (Figure 4). It is noteworthy that these effects pertain to TCR-mediated events. Stimuli that bypass the TCR are less affected or not affected (McDougal, 1988; Klatzmann et al., 1990; McDougal et al., 1991). Immunosuppressive properties have been attributed to other HIV gene products as well (Viscidi et al., 1989; Chanh et al., 1988). These in vitro findings are consistent with clinical features of HIV infection. Antigen specific responses, especially responses to new antigens, tend to be impaired earlier and more profoundly than are responses to nonspecific mitogens and to alloantigens (Clerici et al., 1991; Huang et al., 1987; Lane et al., 1983).

Separate cross-linking of CD4 by monoclonal antibodies before specific, class II MHC-restricted, antigen recognition by the TCR prevents the coclustering of CD4 with the TCR/CD3 complex and can be a potent signal for tolerance (Alters et al., 1990; Merkenschlager et al., 1990; Bank and Chess, 1985; Rosoff et al., 1987). Instead of inducing signal transduction pathways leading to functional activation, programmed cell death or apoptosis occurs. Gp120, attached to CD4 and cross linked by anti-gp120 antibodies, can also prime cells for an apoptotic response after

Immunosuppression Due to gp120 Blocking of CD4: MHC Class II Interaction

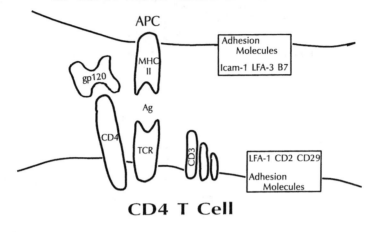

CD4 T Cell

Figure 1.4   Soluble gp120 binds CD4 and may block the amplifying effects of CD4 in the recognition of antigen by the TCR.

TCR recognition (Banda et al., 1992; Terai et al. 1991). Excess apoptotic cells can be detected in HIV–1 infected people (Ameisen, 1992; Groux et al., 1992; Meyaard et al., 1992; Laurent-Crawford et al., 1991). Apoptotic cells are not confined to the CD4 population as might be expected if gp120-primed programmed cell death was the mechanism (Groux et al., 1992; Meyaard et al., 1992; Laurent-Crawford et al., 1991). Moreover, the saturating concentrations of gp120 (or CD4 monoclonal antibody) required to prime cells for apoptosis in vitro are not achieved in blood, though it is possible that they occur transiently in the microenvironment of responding T cells.

Autoimmunity or aberrant immune reactivity

Autoimmune phenomena may occur in the course of HIV infection and have been offered as possible explanations of T cell destruction. Cross-reactions between viral and cellular molecules have been described (Bettaieb et al., 1992; Garry, 1990; Naylor et al., 1987; Parravicini et al.,

1988; Reither et al., 1986; Samuel et al., 1987), particularly cross reactions between regions of HIV envelope and MHC molecules (Atassi and Atassi, 1992; Golding et al., 1988; Golding et al., 1989; Schnittman et al., 1986), and antilymphocyte antibodies with broad cellular reactivity have been reported (Dorsett et al., 1990; Kiprov et al., 1985; Klaassen et al., 1990; Kloster et al., 1984). If these antibodies are important, it is difficult to understand how their broad reactivity results in a selective effect on the CD4 subset. T cell specific autoantibodies have also been described, but there is no apparent correlation between their presence or level and CD4 T cell levels (Stricker et al., 1987; Ardman et al., 1990; Weimer et al., 1991). Antibodies to soluble CD4 are detected in about 10% of HIV infected people (Thiriart et al., 1988; Callahan et al., 1992; Kowalski et al., 1989; Chams et al., 1988; Weimer et al., 1991). They do not react with native CD4 on cell membranes (Callahan et al., 1992; Chams et al., 1988), nor do they bear any relationship to disease severity or CD4 T cell levels (Thiriart et al., 1988; Chams et al., 1988). Finally, the possibility that an antibody response to the binding site of gp120 sets up an idiotypic-anti-idiotypic cascade that ultimately results in anti-CD4 reactive antibodies has theoretical appeal but no practical demonstration (Thiriart et al., 1988; Dreesman and Kennedy, 1985; Karpatkin and Nardi, 1992; Karpatkin et al., 1992).

Several years ago, Zarling and co-workers reported that 11 of 14 HIV-infected patients had non-MHC-restricted cytolytic T cells that recognize uninfected, activated CD4 T cells (Zarling et al., 1990). These cytolytic T cells were not found in uninfected people nor were they found in HIV infected chimpanzees, animals that can be infected but do not develop disease.

Superantigens bind and bridge class II MHC and certain regions of the TCR (Figure 5). Specifically, they bind to relatively invariant regions within the variable region of the TCR beta chain. These invariant regions may be shared within a family of V–beta genes. Depending on the maturation state and microenvironment of the responding T cells, superantigen exposure may result in activation and expansion of CD4 T cells that share expression of the same V–beta gene family; in depletion by induction of apoptosis; or in tolerance induction (anergy). No purified viral protein has been shown, as yet, to have superantigen-like effects in vitro. It is, how-

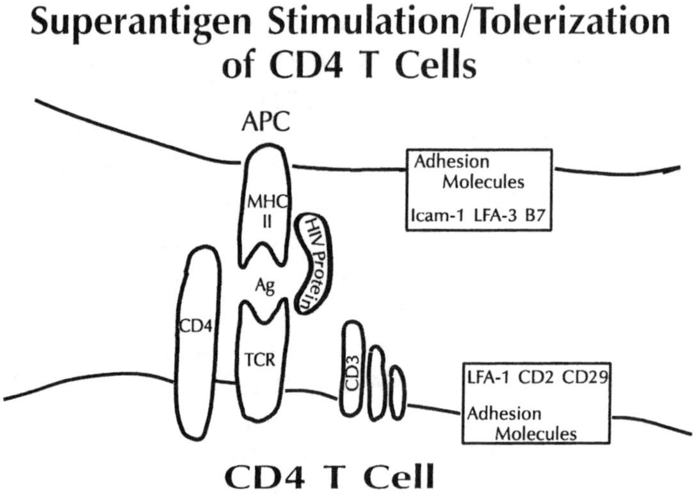

Figure 1.5 Superantigens bind and bridge class II MHC and parts of the TCR not directly involved in antigen contact causing stimulation/tolerance of large subsets (TCR V–beta families) of CD4 T cells.

ever, possible that superantigens from microbial opportunists induce stimulation of T cells subsets, providing a fertile substrate for viral replication. The phenotypic manifestation of a superantigen effect in vivo is the disproportionate expansion or depletion of T cells expressing a particular V–beta gene family or families. Some evidence for depletion of T cells expressing certain V–beta chain families has been reported (Imberti et al., 1991) and T cell clones expressing certain V–beta TCRs may replicate virus better than others (Laurence et al., 1992). Neither of these observations have been confirmed and several studies have failed to detect any phenotypic inference for a superantigen effect in HIV infected people (Dalgleish et al., 1992; Hodara et al., 1993; Posnett et al., 1993; Bisset et al., 1993).

Conclusion

HIV–1 has evolved an affinity for the CD4 molecule and a replication apparatus that is cytopathic for host cells: HIV–1 binds, penetrates, replicates in, and destroys CD4 T cells. Activation and CD4 expression are sufficient and necessary cellular substrates for optimal viral replication and cytopathicity. Numerical/functional depletion of CD4 T cells, progressive viral replication; and inappropriate cellular activation occur over time, resulting in progressive paralysis of immune responsiveness and rendering the infected person susceptible to opportunistic infections and malignancies. Within this framework, much remains to be learned about factors that govern the control and extent of infection. This includes factors that may seem to be only tangentially related to HIV and its effect on CD4 cells: inappropriate and sustained cellular activation, cytokine production, selective pressures governing the evolution of HIV genetic and biologic diversity in the host, immune regeneration in a microenvironment destroyed by HIV, and immune and cellular responses that control rather than compound HIV spread and replication.

References

Albert, J., B. Abramhamsson, K. Nagy, E. Aurelius, H. Gaines, G. Nystrom, and E. M. Fenyo. (1990). Rapid development of isolate-specific neutralizing antibodies after primary HIV-1 infection and consequent emergence of virus variants which resist neutralization by autologous sera. *AIDS 4*:107–112.

Alters, S. E., K. Sakai, L. Steinman, and V. T. Oi. (1990). Mechanisms of anti-CD4-mediated depletion and immunotherapy. *J. Immunol. 144*:4587–4592.

Ameisen, J. C. (1992). Programmed cell death and AIDS: from hypothesis to experiment. *Immunol. Today 13*:388–391.

Ardman, B., M. A. Sikorski, M. Settles, and D. E. Staunton. (1990). Human immunodeficiency virus type 1-infected individuals make autoantibodies that bind to CD43 on normal thymic lymphocytes. *J. Exp. Med. 172*:1151–1158.

Arendrup, M., C. Nielsen, J. E. S. Hansen, C. Pedersen, L. Mathiesen, and J. O. Nielsen. (1992). Autologous HIV-1 neutralizing antibodies: emergence of neutralization-resistant escape virus and subsequent development of escape virus neutralizing antibodies. *J. Acquir. Immune Defic. Syndr. 5*:303–307.

Armstrong, J. A. and R. Horne. (1984). Follicular dendritic cells and virus-like particles in AIDS-related lymphadenopathy. *Lancet 2*:370–372.

Atassi, H. and M. Z. Atassi. (1992). HIV envelope protein is recognized as an alloantigen by human DR-specific alloreactive T cells. *Hum. Immunol. 34*:31–38.

Bagasra, O., S. P. Hauptman, H. W. Lischner, M. Sachs, and R. J. Pomerantz. (1992). Detection of human immunodeficiency virus type 1 provirus in mononuclear cells by in situ polymerase chain reaction. *N. Engl. J. Med. 326*:1385–1391.

Banda, N. K., J. Bernier, D. K. Kurahara, R. Kurrie, N. Haigwood, R. -P. Sekaly, and T. H. Finkel. (1992). Crosslinking CD4 by HIV gp120 primes T cells for activation-induced apoptosis. *J. Exp. Med. 176*:1099–1106.

Bank, I. and L. Chess. (1985). Perturbation of the T4 molecule transmits a negative signal to T cells. *J. Exp. Med. 162*:1294–1303.

Bettaieb, A., P. Fromont, F. Loache, E. Oksenhendler, W. Vainchenker, N. Duedari, and P. Bierling. (1992). Presence of cross–reactive antibody between human immunodeficiency virus (HIV) and platelet glycoproteins in HIV-related immune thrombocytopenic purpura. *Blood 80*:162–169.

Bisset, L. R., M. Opravil, E. Ludwig, and W. Fierz. (1993). T cell response to staphylococcal superantigens by asymptomatic HIV-infected individuals exhibits selective changes in T cell receptor V–beta-chain usage. *AIDS Res. Hum. Retroviruses 9*:241–245.

Boyer, V., C. Desgranges, M-A. Trabaud, E. Fischer, and M. D. Kazatchkine. (1991). Complement mediates human immunodeficiency virus type 1 infection of a human T cell line in a CD4- and antibody-independent fashion. *J. Exp. Med. 173*:1151–1158.

Broder, C. C., D. S. Dimitrov, R. Blumenthal, and E. A. Berger. (1993). The block to HIV-1 envelope glycoprotein-mediated membrane fusion in animal cells expressing human CD4 can be overcome by a human cell component(s). *Virology 193*:483–491.

Callahan, L. N., G. Roderiquez, M. Mallinson, and M. A. Norcross. (1992). Analysis of HIV-induced autoantibodies to cryptic epitopes on human CD4. *J. Immunol. 149*:2194–2202.

Cameron, P. U., P. S. Freudenthal, J. M. Barker, S. Gezelter, K. Inaba, and R. M. Steinman. (1992). Dendritic cells exposed to human immunodeficiency virus type–1 transmit a vigorous cytopathic infection to CD4+ T cells. *Science 257*:383–386.

Cann, A. J., J. A. Zack, A. S. Go, S. J. Arrigo, Y. Koyanagi, P. L. Green, S. Pang, and I. S. Y. Chen. (1990). Human immunodeficiency virus type 1 T-cell tropism is determined by events prior to provirus formation. *J. Virol. 64*:4735–4742.

Cefai, D., P. Debre, M. Kaczorek, T. Idziorek, B. Autran, and G. Bismuth. (1990). Human immunodeficiency virus–1 glycoproteins gp120 and gp160 specifically inhibit the CD3/T cell-antigen receptor phosphoinositide transduction pathway. *J. Clin. Invest. 86*:2117–2124.

Celada, F., C. Cambiaggi, J. Maccari S. Burastero, T. Gregory, E. Patzer, J. Porter, C. McDanal, and T. Matthews. (1990). Antibody raised against soluble CD4–rgp120 complex recognizes the CD4 moiety and blocks membrane fusion without inhibiting CD4-gp120 binding. *J. Exp. Med. 172*:1143–1150.

Chams, V., T. Jouault, E. Fenouillet, J. -C. Gluckman, and D. Klatzmann. (1988). Detection of anti-CD4 autoantibodies in the sera of HIV-infected patients using recombinant soluble CD4 molecules. *AIDS 2*:353–361.

Chanh, T. C., R. C. Kennedy, and P. Kanda. (1988). Synthetic peptides homologous to HIV transmembrane glycoprotein suppress normal human lymphocyte blastogenic response. *Cell. Immunol. 111*:77–86.

Cheng-Mayer, C., J. T. Rutka, M. L. Rosenblum, T. McHugh, D. B. Stites, and J. A. Levy. (1987). Human immunodeficiency virus can productively infect cultured glial cells. *Proc. Natl. Acad. Sci. USA 84*:3526–3530.

Chirmule, N., V. S. Kalyanaraman, N. Oyaizu, H. B. Slade, and S. Pahwa. (1990). Inhibition of functional properties of tetanus antigen-specific T-cell clones by envelope glycoprotein gp120 of human immunodeficiency virus. *Blood 75*:152–159.

Clark, S. J., M. S. Saag, W. D. Decker, S. Campbell-Hill, J. L. Roberson, P. J. Veldkamp, J. C. Kappes, B. H. Hahn, and G. M. Shaw. (1991). High titers of cytopathic virus in plasma of patients with symptomatic primary HIV-1 infection. *N. Engl. J. Med. 324*:954–960.

Clerici, M., C. S. Via, D. R. Luccy, E. Roilides, P. A. Pizzo, and G. M. Shearer. (1991). Functional dichotomy of CD4+ T helper lymphocytes in asymptomatic human immunodeficiency virus infection. *Eur. J. Immunol. 21*:665–670.

Cohen, D. I., Y. Tani, H. Tian, E. Boone, L. W. Samelson, and Lane, E. C. (1992). Participation of tyrosine phosphorylation in the cytopathic effect of human immunodeficiency virus-1. *Science 256*:542–545.

Connor, R. I., N. B. Dinces, A. L. Howell, J. L. Romet-Lemonne, J. L. Pasquali, and M. W. Fanger. (1991). Fc receptors for IgG (FcΓRs) on human monocytes and macrophages are not infectivity receptors for human immunodeficiency virus type 1 (HIV–1): studies using bispecific antibodies to target HIV–1 to various myeloid cell surface molecules, including the FcrR. *Proc. Natl. Acad. Sci. USA 88*:9593–9597.

Connor, R. I., H. Mohri, Y. Cao, and D. D. Ho. (1993). Increased viral burden and cytopathicity correlate temporally with CD4+ T-lymphocyte decline and clinical progression in human immunodeficiency virus type 1-infected individuals. *J. Virol. 67*:1772–1777.

Crise, B. and J. K. Rose. (1992). Human immunodeficiency virus type 1 glycoprotein precursor retains CD4–p56lck complex in the endoplasmic reticulum. *J. Virol. 66*:2296–2301.

Daar, E. S., T. Moudgh, R. D. Meyer, and D. D. Ho. (1991). Transient high levels of viremia in patients with primary human immunodeficiency virus type 1 infection. *N. Engl. J. Med. 324*:961–964.

Dalgleish, A. G., P. C. L. Beverley, P. R. Clapham, D. H. Crawford, M. F. Greaves, and R. A. Weiss. (1984). The CD4 (T4) antigen is an essential component of the receptor for the AIDS retrovirus. *Nature 312*:763–767.

Dalgleish, A. G., S. Wilson, M. Gompels, C. Ludlam, B. Gazzard, A. M. Coates, and J. Habeshaw. (1992). T-cell receptor variable gene products and early HIV infection. *Lancet 339*:824–828.

de Wolf, F., M. Roos, J. M. A. Lange, J. T. M. Houweling, R. A. Coutinho, J. van der Noordaa, P. T. Schellekekns, and J. Goudsmit. (1988). Decline in CD4+ cell numbers reflects increase in HIV–1 replication. *AIDS Res. Hum. Retroviruses 4*:433–439.

Deen, K. C., J. S. McDougal, R. Inacker, C. Golena-Wasserman, J. Arthos, J. Rosenberg, P. J. Maddon, R. Axell, and R. W. Sweet. (1988). A soluble form of CD4 (T4) protein inhibits AIDS virus infection. *Nature 331*:82–84.

DeRossi, A., C. Franchinin, A. Aldorini, A. Del Mistro, A. Chieco-Bianchi, R. C. Gallo, and F. Wong-Staal. (1986). Differential response to the cytopathic effects of human T-cell lymphotropic virus type III (HTLV–III) superinfection in T4+ (helper) and T8+ (suppressor) T cell clones transformed by HTLV–I. *Proc. Natl. Acad. Sci. USA 83*:4297–4301.

Diamond, D. C., B. P. Sleckman, T. Gregory, L. A. Lasky, J. L. Greenstein, and S. J. Burakoff. (1988). Inhibition of CD4+ T cell function by the HIV envelope protein, gp120. *J. Immunol. 141*:3715–3717.

Dorsett, B. H., W. Cronin, and H. L. Loachim. (1990). Presence and prognostic significance of antilymphocyte antibodies in symptomatic and asymptomatic human immunodeficiency virus infection. *Arch. Intern. Med. 150*:1025–1028.

Dragic, T., P. Charneau, F. Clavel, and M. Alizon. (1992). Complementation of murine cells for human immunodeficiency virus envelope/CD4-mediated fusion in human/murine heterokaryons. *J. Virol. 66*:4794–4802.

Dreesmnan, G. R. and R. C. Kennedy. (1985). Anti-idiotypic antibodies: implications of internal image-based vaccines for infectious diseases. *J. Infect. Dis. 151*:761–765.

Dubay, J. W., S. J. Roberts, B. Brody, and E. Hunter. (1992). Mutations in the leucine zipper of the human immunodeficiency virus type 1 transmembrane glycoprotein affect fusion and infectivity. *J. Virol. 66*:4748–4756.

Embretson, J., M. Zupancic, J. L. Ribas, A. Burke, P. Racz, K. Tenner-Racz, and A. T. Haase. (1993). Massive covert infection of helper T lymphocytes and macrophages by HIV during the incubation period of AIDS. *Nature 362*:359–362.

Fauci, A. S. (1993). Multifactorial nature of human immunodeficiency virus disease: implications for therapy. *Science 262*:1011–1018.

Fisher, A. G., E. Collalti, L. Ratner, R. C. Gallo, and F. Wong-Staal. (1985). A molecular clone of HTLV–III with biological activity. *Nature 316*:262–265.

Fisher, R. A., J. M. Bertonis, W. Meier, V. A. Johnson, D. S. Costopoulos, T. Liu, R. Tizard, B. D. Walker, M. S. Hirsch, R. T. Schooley, and R. A. Flavell. (1988). HIV infection is blocked in vitro by recombinant soluble CD4. *Nature 331*:76–78.

Folks, T., J. Kelly, S. Benn, A. Kinter, J. Justement, J. Gold, R. Redfield, K. W. Sell, and A. S. Fauci. (1986a). Susceptibility of normal human lymphocytes to infection with HTLV–III/LAV. *J. Immunol. 136*:4049–4053.

Folks, T., D. M. Powell, M. M. Lightfoote, S. Benn, M. A. Martin, and A. S. Fauci. (1986b). Induction of HTLV–III/LAV from a nonvirus-producing T-cell line: implications for latency. *Science 231*:600–602.

Folks, T. M., K. A. Clouse, J. Justement, A. Rabson, E. Duh, J. H. Kehrl, and A. S. Fauci. (1989). Tumor necrosis factor α induces expression of human immunodeficiency virus in a chronically infected T-cell clone. *Proc. Natl. Acad. Sci. USA 86*:2365–2368.

Gallaher, W. R. (1987). Detection of a fusion peptide sequence in the transmembrane protein of human immunodeficiency virus. *Cell 50*:327–328.

Garcia, J. V. and D. Miller. (1991). Serine phosphorylation-independent downregulation of cell-surface CD4 by *nef*. *Nature 350*:508–511.

Garry, R. F. (1990). Extensive antigenic mimicry by retrovirus capsid proteins. *AIDS Res. Hum. Retroviruses 6*:1361–1362.

Gartner, S., P. Markovits, D. M. Markovitz, M. H. Kaplan, R. C. Gallo, and M. Popovic. (1986). The role of mononuclear phagocytes in HTLV–III/LAV infection. *Science 233*:215–219.

Golding, H., F. A. Robey, F. T. Gates,III, W. Linder, P. R. Beining, T. Hoffman, and B. Golding. (1988). Identification of homologous regions in human immunodeficiency virus I gp41 and human MHC class II β 1 domain. Monoclonal antibodies against the gp41-derived peptide and patients' sera react with native HLA class II antigens, suggesting a role for autoimmunity in the pathogenesis of acquired immune deficiency syndrome. *J. Exp. Med. 167*:914–923.

Golding, H., C. M. Shearer, K. Hillman, P. Lucas, J. Manischewitz, R. A. Zajac, M. Clerici, R. E. Cress, R. N. Boswell, and B. Golding. (1989). Common epitope in human immunodeficiency virus (HIV)–1-gp4l– and HLA class II elicits immunosuppressive autoantibodies capable of contributing to immune dysfunction in HIV–1-infected individuals. *J. Clin. Invest. 83*:1430–1435.

Gotch, F., S. Rowland-Jones, and D. Nixon. (1992). Longitudinal study of HIV-gag specific cytotoxic T lymphocyte responses over time in several patients. *In* P. Racz, N. L. Letvin, and J. C. Gluckman (eds.), *Cytotoxic T cells in HIV and other retroviral infections*. S. Karger, Basel. p. 60–65.

Gowda, S. D., B. S. Stein, N. Mohagheghpour, and C. J. Benike. (1989). Evidence that T cell activation is required for HIV-1 entry in CD4+ lymphocytes. *J. Immunol. 142*:773–780.

Graziosi, C., G. Pantaleo, L. Butini, J. F. Demarest, M. S. Saag, G. M. Shaw, and A. S. Fauci. (1993). Kinetics of human immunodeficiency virus type 1 (HIV–1) DNA and RNA synthesis during primary HIV–1 infection. *Proc. Natl. Acad. Sci. USA 90*:6405–6409.

Gregersen, J. P., S. Mehdi, A. Baur, and J. Hilfenhaus. (1990). Antibody- and complement-mediated lysis of HIV-infected cells and inhibition of viral replication. *J. Med. Virol. 30*:287–293.

Groenink, M., R. A. M. Fouchier, R. E. Y. de Goede, F. de Wolf, R. A. Gruters, H. T. M. Cuypers, H. G. Huisinan, and M. Tersmette. (1991). Phenotypic heterogeneity in a panel of infectious molecular human immunodeficiency virus type 1 clones derived from a single individual. *J. Virol. 65*:1968–1975.

Groux, H., G. Torpier, D. Monté, Y. Mouton, A. Capron, and J. C. Ameisen. (1992). Activation-induced death by apoptosis in CD4 T cells from human immunodeficiency virus-infected asymptomatic individuals. *J. Exp. Med. 175*:331–340.

Guy, B., M. P. Kieny, Y. Riviere, C. Le Peuch, K. Dott, M. Girard, L. Montagnier, and J. -P. Lecocq. (1987). HIV F/3´ orf encodes a phosphorylated GTP-binding protein resembling an oncogene product. *Nature 330*:266–269.

Hahn, B. H., G. M. Shaw, M. E. Taylor, R. R. Redfield, P. D. Markham, S. Z. Salahuddin, F. Wong-Staal, R. C. Gallo, E. S. Parks, and W. P. Parks. (1986). Genetic variation in HTLV–III/LAV over time in patients with AIDS or at risk for AIDS. *Science* 232:1548–1553.

Harouse, J. M., S. Bhat, S. L. Spitalnik, M. Laughlin, K. Stefano, D. H. Silberberg, and F. Gonzalez-Scarano. (1991). Inhibition of entry of HIV–I in neural cell lines by antibodies against galactosyl ceramide. *Science* 253:320–323.

Harper, M. E., L. M. Marselle, R. C. Gallo, and F. Wong-Staal. (1986). Detection of lymphocytes expressing human T-lymphocytotropic virus type III in lymph nodes and peripheral blood from infected individuals by in situ hybridization. *Proc. Natl. Acad. Sci. USA* 83:772–776.

Helseth, E., U. Olshevsky, D. Gabuzda, B. Ardman, W. Haseltine, and J. Sodroski. (1990). Changes in the transmembrane region of the human immunodeficiency virus type 1 gp41 envelope glycoprotein affect membrane fusion. *J. Virol.* 64:6314–6318.

Hodara, V. L., M. Jeddi-Tehrani, J. Grunewald, R. Andersson, G. Scarlatti, S. Esin, V. Holmberg, O. Libonatti, and H. Wigzell. (1993). HIV infection leads to differential expression of T-cell receptor V–beta genes in CD4+ and CD8+ T cells. *AIDS* 7:633–638.

Hofmann, B., P. Nishanian, R. L. Baldwin, P. Insixiengmay, A. Nel, and J. L. Fahey. (1990). HIV inhibits the early steps of lymphocyte activation, including initiation of inositol phopholipid metabolism. *J. Immunol.* 145:3699–3705.

Holmes, E. C., L. Q. Zhang, P. Simmonds, C. A. Ludlam, and A. J. L. Brown. (1992). Convergent and divergent sequence evolution in the surface envelope glycoprotein of human immunodeficiency virus type 1 within a single infected patient. *Proc. Natl. Acad. Sci. USA* 89:4835–4839.

Homsy, J., M. Meyer, and J. A. Levy. (1990). Serum enhancement of human immunodeficiency virus (HIV) correlates with disease in HIV-infected individuals. *J. Virol.* 64:1437–1440.

Homsy, J. M., M. Meyer, M. Tateno, S. Clarkson, and J. A. Levy. (1989). The Fc and not the CD4 receptor mediates antibody enhancement of HIV infection in human cells. *Science* 244:1357–1360.

Horak, I. D., M. Popovic, E. M. Horak, P. J. Lucas, R. E. Gress, C. H. June, and J. B. Bolen. (1990). No T-cell tyrosine protein kinase signalling or calcium mobilization after CD4 association with HIV–1 or HIV–1 gp120. *Nature* 348:557–560.

Hoxie, J. A., J. D. Alpers, J. L. Rackowski, K. Huebner, B. S. Haggarty, A. J. Cedarbaum, and J. C. Reed. (1986). Alterations in T4 (CD4) protein and mRNA synthesis in cells infected with HIV. *Science* 234:1123–1127.

Huang, K. L., F. L. Ruben, C. R. Rinaldo, L. Kingsley, D. W. Lyter, and M. Ho. (1987). Antibody responses after influenza and pneumococcal immunization in HIV-infected homosexual men. *J. Amer. Med. Assoc.* 2577:2047–2050.

Hussey, R. E., N. E. Richardson, M. Kowalski, N. R. Brown, H. -C. Chang, R. F. Siliciano, T. Dorfman, B. Walker, J. Sodroski, and E. L. Reinherz. (1988). A soluble CD4 protein selectively inhibits HIV replication and syncytium formation. *Nature* *331*:78–81.

Imberti, L., A. Sottini, A. Bettinardi, M. Puoti, and D. Primi. (1991). Selective depletion in HIV infection of T cells that bear specific T cell receptor V β-sequences. *Science 254*:860–862.

Jiang, S., K. Lin, and A. R. Neurath. (1991). Enhancement of human immunodeficiency virus type 1 infection by antisera to peptides from the envelope glycoproteins gp120/gp41. *J. Exp. Med. 174*:1557–1563.

Johnson, R. P., A. Trocha, T. M. Buchanan, and B. D. Walker. (1992). Identification of overlapping HLA class I-restricted cytotoxic T cell epitopes in a conserved region of the human immunodeficiency virus type 1 envelope glycoprotein: definition of minimum epitopes and analysis of the effects of sequence variation. *J. Exp. Med. 175*:961–971.

Joling, P., L. J. Bakker, J. A. G. Van Strijp, T. Meerloo, L. de Graaf, M. E. M. Dekker, J. Goudsmit, J. Verhoef, and H. -J. Schuurman. (1993). Binding of human immunodeficiency virus type-1 to follicular dendritic cells in vitro is complement dependent. *J. Immunol. 150*:1065–1073.

Joualt, T., F. Chapuis, R. Olivier, C. Parravicini, E. Bahraoui, and J. -C. Gluckiman. (1989). HIV infection of monocytic cells: role of antibody-mediated virus binding to Fc-gamma receptors. *AIDS 3*:125–133.

Karpatkin, S. and M. Nardi. (1992). Autoimmune anti-HIV–1 gp120 antibody with antiidiotype-like activity in sera and immune complexes of HIV–1-related immunologic thrombocytopenia. *J. Clin. Invest. 89*:356–364.

Karpatkin, S., M. A. Nardi, and Y. H. Kouri. (1992). Internal image anti-idiotype HIV–1 gp120 antibody in human immunodeficiency virus 1 (HIV–1)-seropositive individuals with thrombocytopenia. *Proc. Natl. Acad. Sci. USA 89*:1487–1491.

Kiprov, D. D., R. E. Anderson, P. R. Morand, D. M. Simpson, J. -C. Chermann, J. A. Levy, and A. R. Moss. (1985). Antilymphocyte antibodies and seropositivity for retroviruses in groups at high risk for AIDS. *N. Engl. J. Med. 312*:1517.

Klaassen, R. J. L., J. W. Mulder, A. B. J. Vlekke, J. K. M. Eeftinck Schattenkerk, H. M. Weigel, J. M. A. Lange, and A. E. G. K. von dem Borne. (1990). Autoantibodies against peripheral blood cells appear early in HIV infection and their prevalence increases with disease progression. *Clin. Exp. Immunol. 81*:11–17.

Klatzmann, D., E. Champagne, S. Chamaret, J. Gruest, D. Guetard, T. Hercend, J. -C. Gluckman, and L. Montagnier. (1984). T-lymphocyte T4 molecule behaves as the receptor for human retrovirus LAV. *Nature 312*:767–768.

Klatzmann, D. R., J. S. McDougal, and P. J. Maddon. (1990). The CD4 molecule and HIV infection. *Immunodefic. Rev. 23*:43–66.

Kloster, B. E., R. H. Tomar, and T. J. Spira. (1984). Lymphocytotoxic antibodies in the acquired immunodeficiency syndrome (AIDS). *Clin. Immunol. Immunopathol. 30*:330–335.

Koenig, S., H. E. Gendelman, J. M. Orenstein, M. C. D. Canto, G. H. Kezeshkpour, M. Yungbluth, F. Janotta, A. Aksamit, M. A. Martin, and A. S. Fauci. (1986). Detection of AIDS virus in macrophages in brain tissue from AIDS patients with ence-phalophathy. *Science 233*:1089–1093.

Koga, Y., M. Sasaki, K. Nakamura, G. Kimura, and K. Nomoto. (1990). Intracellular distribution of the envelope glycoprotein of human immunodeficiency virus and its role in the production of cytopathic effect in CD4+ and CD4- human cell lines. *J. Virol. 64*:4661–4671.

Koga, Y., M. Sasaki, H. Yoshida, M. Oh-Tsu, G. Kimura, and K. Nomoto. (1991). Disturbance of nuclear transport of proteins in CD4+ cells expressing gp160 of human immunodeficiency virus. *J. Virol. 65*:5609–5612.

Koot, M., I. P. M. Keet, A. H. V. Vos, R. E. Y. de Goede, M. T. L. Roos, R. A. Coutino, F. Miedema, P. T. A. Schellekens, and M. Tersmette. (1993). Prognostic value of HIV-1 syncytium-inducing phenotype for rate of CD4+ cell depletion and progression to AIDS. *Ann. Intern. Med. 118*:681–688.

Kowalski, M., B. Ardman, L. Basiripour, Y. Lu, D. Blohm, W. Haseltine, and J. Sodroski. (1989). Antibodies to CD4 in individuals infected with human immunodeficiency virus type 1. *Proc. Natl. Acad. Sci. USA 86*:3346–3350.

Kowalski, M., J. Potz, L. Basiripour, T. Dorfman, W. C. Goh, E. Terwilliger, A. Dayton, C. Rosen, W. Haseltine, and J. Sodroski. (1987). Functional regions of the envelope glycoprotein of human immunodeficiency virus type 1. *Science 237*:1351–1355.

Kuiken, C. L., J. -J. De Jong, E. Baan, W. Keulen, M. Tersmette, and J. Goudsmit. (1992). Evolution of the V3 envelope domain in proviral sequences and isolates of human immunodeficiency virus type 1 during transition of the viral biological phenotype. *J. Virol. 66*:4622–4627.

Lane, H. C., H. Masur, L. C. Edgar, G. Whalen, A. H. Rook, and A. S. Fauci. (1983). Abnormalities of B cell activation and immunoregulation in patients with the acquired immunodeficiency syndrome. *N. Engl. J. Med. 309*:453–458.

Lanzavecchia, A., E. Roosnek, T. Gregory, P. Berman, and S. Abrignani. (1988). T cells can present antigens such as HIV gp120 targeted to their own surface molecules. *Nature 334*:530–534.

Laurence, J., A. S. Hodstev, and D. N. Posnett. (1992). Superantigen implicated in dependence of HIV-1 replication in T cells on TCR VB expression. *Nature 358*:255–259.

Laurent-Crawford, A. G., B. Krust, S. Muller, Y. Riviere, M. -A. Rey-Cuille, J. -M. Bechet, L. Montagnier, and A. G. Hovanessian. (1991). The cytopathic effect of HIV is associated with apoptosis. *Virology 185*:829–839.

Levy, J. A. (1993). Pathogenesis of human immunodeficiency virus infection. *Microbiol. Rev. 57*:183–289.

Levy, J. A., C. Cheng-Mayer, D. Dina, and P. A. Luciw. (1986). AIDS retrovirus (ARV-2) clone replicates in transfected human and animal fibroblasts. *Science 232*:998–1001.

Li, X. L., T. Moudgil, H. V. Vinters, and D. D. Ho. (1990). CD4-independent, productive infection of a neuronal cell line by human immunodeficiency virus type 1. *J. Virol. 64*:1383–1387.

Lifson, J. D., M. B. Feinberg, G. R. Reyes, L. Rabin, B. Banapour, S. Chakrabarti, B. Moss, F. Wong-Staal, K. S. Steirner, and E. G. Engleman. (1986a). Induction of CD4-dependent cell fusion by the HTLV–III/LAV envelope glycoprotein. *Nature 323*:725–728.

Lifson, J. D., G. R. Reyes, M. S. McGrath, B. S. Stein, and E. G. Engleman. (1986b). AIDS retrovirus induced cytopathology: giant cell formation and involvement of CD4 antigen. *Science 232*:1123–1127.

Linette, G. P., R. J. Hartzman, J. A. Ledbetter, and C. H. June. (1988). HIV–1-infected T cells show a selective signaling defect after perturbation of CD3/antigen receptor. *Science 241*:573–576.

Ljunggren, K., B. Böttinger, G. Biberfeld, A. Karlson, E. -M. Fenyö, and M. Jondal. (1987). Antibody-dependent cellular cytotoxicity-inducing antibodies against human immunodeficiency virus. *J. Immunol. 139*:2263–2267.

Mackewicz, C. E., H. W. Ortega, and J. A. Levy. (1991). CD8+ cell anti-HIV activity correlates with the clinical state of the infected individual. *J. Clin. Invest. 87*:1462–1466.

Maddon, P. J., A. G. Dalgleish, J. S. McDougal, P. R. Clapham, R. A. Weiss, and R. Axel. (1986). The T4 gene encodes the AIDS virus receptor and is expressed in the immune system and the brain. *Cell 47*:333–348.

Maddon, P. J., J. S. McDougal, P. R. Clapham, A. G. Dalgleish, S. Jamal, R. A. Weiss, and R. Axel. (1988). HIV infection does not require endocytosis of its receptor, CD4. *Cell 54*:865–874.

Marsh, M. and A. Dalgleish. (1987). How do human immunodeficiency viruses enter cells? *Immunol. Today 8*:369–371.

McDougal, J. S. (1988). Function of the CD4 molecule in normal immune responses. *Curr. Opin. Immunol. 1*:88–91.

McDougal, J. S., M. S. Kennedy, J. K. A. Nicholson, T. J. Spira, H. W. Jaffe, J. E. Kaplan, D. B. Fishbein, P. O'Malley, C. Aloisio, C. M. Black, M. Hubbard, and C. B. Reimer. (1987). Antibody response to human immunodeficiency virus in homosexual men. Relation of antibody specificity, titer, and isotype to clinical status, severity of immunodeficiency and disease progression. *J. Clin. Invest. 80*:316–324.

McDougal, J. S., M. S. Kennedy, J. M. Sligh, S. P. Cort, A. Mawle, and J. K. A. Nicholson. (1986a). Binding of HTLV–III/LAV to T4+ T cells by a complex of the 110K viral protein and the T4 molecule. *Science 231*:382–385.

McDougal, J. S., D. R. Klatzmann, and P. J. Maddon. (1991). CD4–gp120 interactions. *Curr. Opin. Immunol. 3*:552–558.

McDougal, J. S., A. Mawle, S. P. Cort, J. K. A. Nicholson, G. D. Cross, J. A. Scheppler-Campbell, D. Hicks, and J. Sligh. (1985). Cellular tropism of the human retrovirus HTLV–III/LAV. Role of T cell activation and expression of the T4 antigen. *J. Immunol. 135*:3151–3162.

McDougal, J. S., J. K. A. Nicholson, G. D. Cross, S. P. Cort, M. S. Kennedy, and A. C. Mawle. (1986b). Binding of the human retrovirus HTLV–III/LAV/ARV/HIV to the CD4 (T4) molecule: conformation dependence, epitope mapping, antibody inhibition, and potential for idiotypic mimicry. *J. Immunol. 137*:2937–2944.

McKeating, J. A., P. D. Griffiths, and R. A. Weiss. (1990). HIV susceptibility conferred to human fibroblasts by cytomegalovirus-induced Fc receptor. *Nature 343*:659–661.

Merkenschlager, M., D. Buck, P. C. L. Beverley, and Q. J. Sattentau. (1990). Functional epitope analysis of the human CD4 molecule. The MHC class II-dependent activation of resting T cells is inhibited by monoclonal antibodies to CD4 regardless of whether or not they recognize epitopes involved in the binding of MHC class II or HIV gp120. *J. Immunol. 145*:2839–2845.

Meyaard, L., S. A. Otto, R. R. Jonker, M. J. Mijnster, R. P. M. Keet, and F. Miedema. (1992). Programmed death of T cells in HIV–1 infection. *Science 257*:217–219.

Mittler, R. S. and M. K. Hoffmann. (1989). Synergism between HIV gp120 and gp120-specific antibody in blocking human T cell activation. *Science 245*:1380–1382.

Montefiori, D. C., M. Murphey-Corb, R. C. Desrosiers, and M. D. Daniel. (1990). Complement-mediated, infection-enhancing antibodies in plasma from vaccinated macaques before and after inoculation with live simian immunodeficiency virus. *J. Virol. 64*:5223–5225.

Moore, J. P., Q. J. Sattentau, P. J. Kiasse, and L. C. Burkly. (1992). A monoclonal antibody to CD4 domain 2 blocks soluble CD4-induced conformational changes in the envelope glycoproteins of human immunodeficiency virus type 1 (HIV–1) and HIV–1 infection of CD4+ cells. *J. Virol. 66*:4784–4793.

Naylor, P. H., C. W. Naylor, M. Badamchian, S. Wada, A. L. Goldstein, S. -S. Wang, D. K. Sun, A. H. Thornton, and P. S. Sarin. (1987). Human immunodeficiency virus contains an epitope immunoreactive with thymosin alpha–1 and the 30–amino acid synthetic p17 group-specific antigen peptide HGP–30. *Proc. Natl. Acad. Sci. USA 84*:2951–2955.

Nicholson, J. K. A., G. D. Cross, C. S. Callaway, and J. S. McDougal. (1986). In vitro infection of human monocytes with human T lymphotropic virus type III/lymphadenopathy-associated virus (HTLV–III/LAV). *J. Immunol. 137*:323–329.

Nicholson, J. K. A., B. M. Jones, D. F. Echenberg, T. J. Spira, and J. S. McDougal. (1987). Phenotypic distribution of T cells of patients who have subsequently developed AIDS. *Clin. Immunol. Immunopath. 43*:82–87.

Nicholson, J. K. A., J. S. McDougal, T. J. Spira, G. D. Cross, B. M. Jones, and E. L. Reinherz. (1984). Immunoregulatory subsets of the T helper and T suppressor cell populations in homosexual men with chronic unexplained lymphadenopathy. *J. Clin. Invest. 73*:191–201.

Nixon, D. F., A. R. M. Townsend, J. G. Elvin, C. R. Rizza, J. Galiwey, and A. J. McMichael. (1988). HIV–1 gag-specific cytotoxic T lymphocytes defined with recombinant vaccinia virus and synthetic peptides. *Nature 336*:484–487.

Orentas, R. J., J. E. K. Hudreth, E. Obah, M. Polydefkis, C. E. Smith, N. L. Clements, and R. F. Siliciano. (1990). Induction of CD4+ human cytolytic T cells specific for HIV-infected cells by a gp160 subunit vaccine. *Science 248*:1234–1237.

Orloff, C. N., N. S. Kennedy, C. Dawson, and J. S. McDougal. (1991a). HIV–1 binding to CD4 T cells does not induce a Ca$2+$ influx or lead to activation of protein kinases. *AIDS Res. Hum. Retroviruses* 7:587–593.

Orloff, C. M., S. L. Orloff, M. S. Kennedy, P. J. Maddon, and J. S. McDougal. (1991b). Penetration of CD4 T cells by HIV–1. The CD4 receptor does not internalize with HIV, and CD4-related signal transduction events are not required for entry. *J. Immunol.* 146:2578–2587.

Oyaizu, N., N. Chirmule, V. S. Kalyanaraman, W. W. Hall, R. A. Good, and S. Pahwa. (1990). Human immunodeficiency virus type 1 envelope glycoprotein gp120 produces immune defects in CD4$^+$ T lymphocytes by inhibiting interleukin 2 mRNA. *Proc. Natl. Acad. Sci. USA* 87:2379–2383.

Pahwa, S., R. Pahwa, C. Saxinger, R. C. Gallo, and R. A. Good. (1985). Influence of the human T-lymphotropic virus/lymphadenopathy-associated virus on functions of human lymphocytes: evidence for immunosuppressive effects and polyclonal B-cell activation by banded viral preparations. *Proc. Natl. Acad. Sci. USA* 82:8198–8202.

Panteleo, C., C. Graziosi, L. Butini, P. A. Pizzo, S. M. Schnittman, D. P. Kotler, and A. S. Fauci. (1991). Lymphoid organs function as major reservoirs for human immunodeficiency virus. *Proc. Natl. Acad. Sci. USA* 88:9838–9842.

Panteleo, C., C. Graziosi, J. F. Demarest, L. Butini, M. Montroni, C. H. Fox, J. M. Orenstein, D. P. Kotler, and A. S. Fauci. (1993). HIV infection is active and progressive in lymphoid tissue during the clinically latent stage of disease. *Nature* 362:355–358.

Parravicini, C. L., D. Klatzmann, P. Jaffray, G. Costanzi, and J. -C. Gluckman. (1988). Monoclonal antibodies to the human immunodeficiency virus p18 protein cross-react with normal human tissues. *AIDS* 2:171–177.

Perez, L. G., M. A. O'Donnell, and E. B. Stephens. (1992). The transmembrane glycoprotein of human immunodeficiency virus type 1 induces syncytium formation in the absence of the receptor binding glycoprotein. *J. Virol.* 66:4134–4143.

Perno, C. -F., M. W. Baseler, S. Broder, and R. Yarchoan. (1990). Infection of monocytes by human immunodeficiency virus type 1 blocked by inhibitors of CD4–gp120 binding, even in the presence of enhancing antibodies. *J. Exp. Med.* 171:1043–1056.

Phillips, R. E., S. Rowland-Jones, D. F. Nixon, F. M. Gotch, J. P. Edwards, A. O. Ogunlesi, J. G. Elvin, J. A. Rothbard, C. R. M. Bangham, C. R. Rizza, and A. J. McMichael. (1991). Human immunodeficiency virus genetic variation that can escape cytotoxic T cell recognition. *Nature* 354:453–459.

Plata, F., B. Autran, L. Pedroza Martins, S. Wain-Hobson, M. Raphael, C. Nayaud, M. Denis, J. -M. Guillon, and P. Debre. (1987). AIDS virus-specific cytotoxic T lymphocytes in lung disorders. *Nature* 328:348–351.

Polydefkis, M., S. Koenig, C. Flexner, E. Obah, K. Gebo, S. Chakrabarti, P. L. Earl, B. Moss, and R. F. Siliciano. (1990). Anchor sequence-dependent endogenous processing of human immunodeficiency virus 1 envelope glycoprotein gp160 for CD4$^+$ T cell recognition. *J. Exp. Med.* 171:875–887.

Posnett, D. N., S. Kabak, A. S. Hodtsev, E. A. Goldberg, and A. Asch. (1993). T-cell antigen receptor V–beta subsets are not preferentially deleted in AIDS. *AIDS* 7:625–631.

Poulin, L., L. A. Evans, S. Tang, A. Barboza, H. Legg, D. R. Littman, and J. A. Levy. (1991). Several CD4 domains can play a role in human immunodeficiency virus infection of cells. *J. Virol.* 65:4893–4901.

Qureshi, N. M., D. H. Coy, R. F. Garry, and L. A. Henderson. (1990). Characterization of a putative cellular receptor for HIV–1 transmembrane glycoprotein using synthetic peptides. *AIDS* 4:553–558.

Reither, W. E. I., J. E. Blalock, and T. K. Brunck. (1986). Sequence homology between acquired immunodeficiency syndrome virus envelope protein and interleukin 2. *Proc. Natl. Acad. Sci. USA* 83:9188–9192.

Robinson, W. E., D. C. Montefiori, and W. M. Mitchell. (1988). Antibody-dependent enhancement of human immunodeficiency virus type 1 infection. *Lancet 1*:790–794.

Roos, M. T. L., J. M. A. Lange, R. E. Y. de Goede, R. A. Coutino, P. T. A. Schellekens, F. Miedema, and M. Tersmette. (1992). Viral phenotype and immune response in primary human immunodeficiency virus type 1 infection. *J. Infect. Dis.* 165:427–432.

Rosoff, P. M., S. J. Burakoff, and J. L. Greenstein. (1987). The role of the L3T4 molecule in mitogen and antigen-activated signal transduction. *Cell 49*:845–853.

Ruscetti, F. W., J. A. Mikovits, V. S. Kalyanaraman, R. Overton, H. Stevenson, K. Stromberg, R. B. Herberman, W. L. Farrar, and J. R. Ortaldo. (1986). Analysis of effector mechanisms against HTLV–1- and HTLV–III/LAV-infected lymphoid cells. *J. Immunol.* 136:3619–3624.

Saag, M. S., B. H. Hahn, J. Gibbons, Y. Li, E. S. Parks, W. P. Parks, and G. M. Shaw. (1988). Extensive variation of human immunodeficiency virus type–1 *in vivo*. *Nature 334*:440–444.

Samuel, K. P., A. Seth, A. Konopka, J. A. Lautenberger, and T. S. Papas. (1987). The 3′–orf protein of human immunodeficiency virus shows structural homology with the phosphorylation domain of human interleukin–2 receptor and the ATP-binding site of the protein kinase family. *FEBS Lett.* 218:81–86.

Schnittman, S. M., J. J. Greenhouse, M. C. Psallidopoulos, M. Baseler, N. P. Salzman, A. S. Fauci, and H. C. Lane. (1990a). Increasing viral burden in CD4⁺ T cells from patients with human immunodeficiency virus (HIV) infection reflects rapidly progressive immunosuppression and clinical disease. *Ann. Intern. Med. 113*:438–443.

Schnittman, S. M., H. C. Lane, J. Greenhouse, J. S. Justement, M. Baseler, and A. S. Fauci. (1990b). Preferential infection of CD4⁺ memory T cells by human immunodeficiency virus type 1: evidence for a role in the selective T-cell functional defects observed in infected individuals. *Proc. Natl. Acad. Sci. USA* 87:6058–6062.

Schnittman, S. M., H. C. Lane, S. E. Higgins, T. Folks, and A. S. Fauci. (1986). Direct polyclonal activation of human B lymphocytes by the acquired immune deficiency syndrome virus. *Science 233*:1084–1086.

Schnittman, S. M., M. C. Psallidopoulos, H. C. Lane, L. Thompson, M. Baseler, F. Massari, C. H. Fox, N. P. Saizinan, and A. S. Fauci. (1989). The reservoir for HIV-1 in human peripheral blood is a T cell that maintains expression of CD4. *Science* 245:305–308.

Schuitemaker, H., M. Koot, M. A. Kootstra, M. W. Derksen, R. E. De Goede, R. P. Van Steenwijk, J. M. A. Lange, J. K. M. Eeftink Schattenkerk, F. Miedema, and M. Tersmette. (1992). Biological phenotype of human immunodeficiency virus type 1 clones at different stages of infection: progression of disease is associated with a shift from monocytotropic to T-cell-tropic virus populations. *J. Virol.* 66:1354–1360.

Sharer, L. R., C. Eun-Sook, and L. C. Epstein. (1985). Multinucleated giant cells and HTLV-III in AIDS encephalopathy. *Hum. Pathol.* 16:760.

Siliciano, R. F., T. Lawton, C. Knall, R. W. Karr, P. Berman, T. Gregory, and E. L. Reinherz. (1988). Analysis of host–virus interactions in AIDS with anti–gp120 T cell clones: effect of HIV sequence variation and mechanism for CD4+ cell depletion. *Cell* 54:561–575.

Siliciano, R. F., C. Knall, T. Lawton, P. Berman, T. Gregory, and E. L. Reinherz. (1989). Recognition of HIV glycoprotein gp120 by T cells. Role of monocyte CD4 in the presentation of gp120. *J. Immunol.* 142:1506–1511.

Smith, D. H., R. A. Byrn, S. A. Marsters, T. Gregory, J. E. Groopman, and D. J. Capon. (1987). Blocking of HIV-1 infectivity by a soluble, secreted form of the CD4 antigen. *Science* 238:1704–1707.

Sodroski, J., W. C. Goh, C. Rosen, K. Campbell, and W. A. Haseltine. (1986). Role of the HTLV–III/LAV envelope in syncytium formation and cytopathicity. *Nature* 322:470–474.

Spear, G. T., B. L. Sullivan, A. L. Landay, and T. F. Lint. (1990). Neutralization of human immunodeficiency virus type 1 by complement occurs by viral lysis. *J. Virol.* 64:5869–5873.

Spear, C. T., D. M. Taketman, B. L. Sullivan, A. L. Landay, and S. Zolla-Pazner. (1993). Complement activation by human monoclonal antibodies to human immunodeficiency virus. *J. Virol.* 67:53–59.

Stein, B. S., S. D. Gowda, J. D. Lifson, R. C. Penhallow, K. C. Bensch, and E. C. Engleman. (1987). pH-independent HIV entry into CD4-positive T cells via virus envelope fusion to the plasma membrane. *Cell* 49:659–668.

Stricker, R. B., T. M. McHugh, D. J. Moody, W. J. W. Morrow, D. P. Stites, M. A. Shuman, and J. A. Levy. (1987). An AIDS-related cytotoxic autoantibody reacts with a specific antigen on stimulated CD4+ T cells. *Nature* 327:710–713.

Takahashi, H., J. Cohen, A. Hosmalin, K. B. Cease, R. Houghten, J. L. Cornette, C. DeLisi, B. Moss, R. N. Germain, and J. A. Berzofsky. (1988). An immunodominant epitope of the human immunodeficiency virus envelope glycoprotein gp160 recognized by class I major histocompatibility complex molecule-restricted murine cytotoxic T lymphocytes. *Proc. Natl. Acad. Sci. USA* 85:3105–3109.

Takahashi, H., R. Houghten, S. D. Putney, D. H. Margulies, B. Moss, R. N. Germain, and J. A. Berzofsky. (1989). Structural requirements for class I MHC molecule-mediated antigen presentation and cytotoxic T cell recognition of an immunodominant determinant of the human immunodeficiency virus envelope protein. *J. Exp. Med. 170*:2023–2035.

Takeda, A., C. U. Tuazon, and F. A. Ennis. (1988). Antibody-enhanced infection by HIV–1 via Fc receptor-mediated entry. *Science 242*:580–583.

Takeda, A., R. W. Sweet, and F. A. Ennis. (1990). Two receptors are required for antibody-dependent enhancement of human immunodeficiency virus type 1 infection: CD4 and FcΓR. *J. Virol. 64*:5605–5610.

Terai, C., R. S. Kornbluth, C. D. Pauza, D. D. Richman, and D. A. Carson. (1991). Apoptosis as a mechanism of cell death in cultured T lymphoblasts acutely infected with HIV–1. *J. Clin. Invest. 87*:1710–1715.

Thali, M., U. Olshevsky, C. Furman, D. Gabuzda, J. Li, and J. Sodroski. (1991). Effects of changes in gp120–CD4 binding affinity on human immunodeficiency virus type 1 envelope glycoprotein function and soluble CD4 sensitivity. *J. Virol. 65*:5007–5012.

Thiriart, C., J. Goudsmit, P. Schellekens, F. Barin, D. Zagury, M. De Wilde, and C. Bruck. (1988). Antibodies to soluble CD4 in HIV–1-infected individuals. *AIDS 2*:345–351.

Tong-Starksen, S. E., P. A. Luciw, and B. M. Peterlin. (1989). Signaling through T lymphocyte surface proteins TCR/CD3 and CD28, activates the HIV–1 long terminal repeat. *J. Immunol. 142*:702–707.

Traunecker, A., W. Lüke, and K. Karjalainen. (1988). Soluble CD4 molecules neutralize human immunodeficiency virus type 1. *Nature 331*:84–86.

Tremblay, M., and M. A. Wainberg. (1990). Neutralization of multiple HIV–1 isolates from a single subject by autologous sequential sera. *J. Infect. Dis. 162*:735–737.

Truneh, A., D. Buck, D. R. Cassatt, R. Juszczak, S. Kassis, S. -E. Ryu, D. Healey, R. Sweet, and Q. Sattentau. (1991). A region in domain 1 of CD4 distinct from the primary gp120 binding site is involved in HIV infection and virus-mediated fusion. *J. Biol. Chem. 266*:5942–5948.

van Noesel, C. J. M., R. A. Gruters, F. C. Terpstra, P. T. A. Schellekens, R. A. W. van Lier, and F. Miedema. (1990). Functional and phenotypic evidence for a selective loss of memory T cells in asymptomatic human immunodeficiency virus-infected men. *J. Clin. Invest. 86*:293–299.

Viscidi, R. P., K. Mayur, H. M. Lederman, and A. D. Frankel. (1989). Inhibition of antigen-induced lymphocyte proliferation by tat protein from HIV–1. *Science 246*:1606–1608.

Wahl, S. M., J. B. Allen, S. Gartner, J. M. Ornstein, M. Popovic, D. E. Chenowith, L. O. Arthur, W. L. Farrar, and L. M. Wahl. (1989). HIV–1 and its envelope glycoprotein down-regulate chemotactic ligand receptors and chemotactic function of peripheral blood monocytes. *J. Immunol. 142*:3553–3559.

Walker, B. D., S. Chakrabarti, B. Moss, T. J. Paradis, T. Flynn, A. G. Durno, R. S. Blumberg, J. C. Kaplan, M. S. Hirsch, and R. T. Schooley. (1987). HIV-specific cytotoxic T lymphocytes in seropositive individuals. *Nature 328*:345–348.

Weimer, R., V. Daniel, R. Zimmermann, K. Schimpf, and G. Opelz. (1991). Autoantibodies against CD4 cells are associated with CD4 helper defects in human immunodeficiency virus-infected patients. *Blood 77*:133–140.

Weinhold, K. J., H. K. Lyerly, T. J. Matthews, D. S. Tyler, P. M. Ahearne, K. C. Stine, A. J. Langlois, D. T. Durack, and D. P. Bolognesi. (1988). Cellular anti-gp120 cytolytic reactivities in HIV–1 seropositive individuals. *Lancet 1*:902–905.

Weinhold, K. J., H. K. Lyerly, S. D. Stanley, A. A. Austin, T. J. Matthews, and D. P. Bolognesi. (1989). HIV–1 gp120-mediated immune suppression and lymphocyte destruction in the absence of viral infection. *J. Immunol. 142*:3091–3097.

Willey, R. L., F. Maldarelli, M. A. Martin, and K. Strebel. (1992). Human immunodeficiency virus type 1 vpu protein induces rapid degradation of CD4. *J. Virol. 66*:7193–7200.

Willey, R. L., R. A. Rutledge, S. Dias, T. Folks, T. Theodore, C. E. Buckler, and M. A. Martin. (1986). Identification of conserved and divergent domains within the envelope gene of the acquired immunodeficiency syndrome retrovirus. *Proc. Natl. Acad. Sci. USA 83*:5038–5042.

Zack, J. A., S. J. Arrigo, S. R. Weitsman, A. S. Go, A. Haislip, and I. S. Y. Chen. (1990). HIV–1 entry into quiescent primary lymphocytes: molecular analysis reveals a labile, latent viral structure. *Cell 61*:213–222.

Zaqury, D., J. Bernard, R. Leonard, R. Cheynier, M. Feldman, P. S. Sarin, and R. C. Gallo. (1986). Long-term cultures of HTLV–III-infected T cells: a model of cytopathology of T-cell depletion in AIDS. *Science 231*:850–853.

Zarling, J. M., J. A. Ledbetter, J. Sias, P. Fultz, J. Eichborg, G. Gjerset, and P. A. Moran. (1990). HIV-infected humans, but not chimpanzees, have circulating cytotoxic T lymphocytes that lyse uninfected CD4+ cells. *J. Immunol. 144*:2992–2998.

2

Latency and activation of lentiviruses: studies of visna virus in monocytes and macrophages

Janice E. Clements
Department of Comparative Medicine
and Department of Molecular Biology & Genetics
Johns Hopkins University School of Medicine
720 Rutland Avenue, Traylor G–60
Baltimore Maryland 21205, USA

Lucy M. Carruth
Department of Comparative Medicine
Johns Hopkins University School of Medicine

Susan L. Gdovin
Department of Microbiology
University of Maryland
College Park, Maryland 20742, USA

Introduction

The lentiviruses comprise a subfamily of retroviruses that include HIV–1, the causative agent of AIDS (Narayan & Clements, 1990). Lentiviruses cause chronic progressive diseases and the animal lentiviruses have served as models of human diseases such as multiple sclerosis, inflammatory arthritis and interstitial pneumonitis (Narayan & Clements, 1989).

Table 2.1. *Lentiviruses*

Immunodeficiency[a]
Human Immunodeficiency Virus (HIV)
Simian Immunodeficiency Virus (SIV)
Bovine Immunodeficiency Virus (BIV)
Feline Immunodeficiency Virus (FIV)

Lymphoproliferative Disease/Anemia[b]
Visna Virus
Caprine-Arthritis Encephalitis (CAEV)
Equine Infectious Anemia (EIAV)

[a]Viruses have cell tropisms for lymphocytes and macrophage
[b]Viruses have a cell tropism for macrophages

This group of viruses share biological properties and as the name—lenti-virus suggests, they all cause slow infections characterized by a relatively long period between the acute stage of virus infection and manifestation of clinical disease. The common biological features include virus morphology (asymmetric core), replication in non-dividing cells, infection of cells of the immune system, antigenic variation and high level of genetic diversity. The lentiviruses can be separated into viruses that cause immunodeficiency diseases and those that produce lymphoproliferative diseases or anemia (Table 1). One of the differences between the two groups of viruses is that the immunodeficiency viruses have a cell tropism for both T cells and macrophages, whereas the other viruses, the non-primate lentiviruses in general, have cell tropisms limited to monocytes and macrophages. In both cases, the infection of cells of the immune system is central to the production of disease by these viruses.

Lentiviruses cause multi-organ disease that includes infection of lymph nodes, lung, joints and the central nervous system (CNS) (Narayan 1983; Narayan & Clements, 1989). Infection of a host with a lentivirus is characterized by an acute phase of infection (1–4 weeks) that is accompanied

HIV

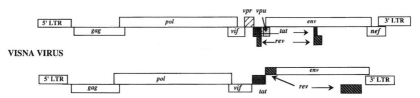

VISNA VIRUS

Figure 1   The genetic organization of two prototype lentiviruses. The HIV DNA is a representative of the immunodeficiency viruses with a more complex array of regulatory genes. Visna virus DNA is representative of the other lentiviruses with a smaller number of regulatory genes, the lack of a distinct *nef*-ORF and the position of the first exon of *rev* is in the same frame as the *env* gene.

by detectable virus replication in the peripheral blood and immune responses (Figure 1). In animal studies, the immune response is rarely effective in eliminating or controlling the virus infection or virally-infected cells. After the acute phase of infection a "latent period" has been described. However, during this period lentiviruses can be found replicating in target organs that include the lymph node, spleen, lung, brain and infected precursor cells can be found in the bone marrow. Thus, this is a period of subclinical infection when virus is highly associated with cells and organs, and virus replication is sequestered in tissues.

The acute phase of infection induces both humoral and cell-mediated immune responses. In the case of the humoral immune response, neutralizing antibodies against the virus are effective in neutralizing the initial virus but the presence of such antibody leads to antigenic drift of the virus *in vivo* (Clements et al., 1988). Neutralizing antibody alone has been shown to select antigenic variants *in vitro* in both the visna virus and EIAV systems. The selection of antigenic variants within a single infected host occurs rapidly due to the high intrinsic mutation rate of these viruses. The intrinsic error rate and lack of editing function of the reverse transcriptase enzyme that transcribes the RNA genome into DNA is the basis of this high mutation rate. The presence of neutralizing antibodies drives the selection of viruses that are not neutralized by the existing antibodies. Changes in the envelope gene of the viruses are responsible for the anti-

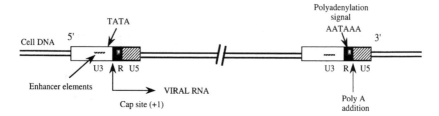

Figure 2   Transcription of lentiviruses is controlled by sequences in the 5′ LTR. The location of important regulatory signals are indicated.

genic changes in visna virus and EIAV, (Clements et al., 1988). There is also a great deal of genetic heterogeneity observed *in vivo* without immune selection as in the case of CAEV (Roberson et al., 1982; Chiu et al., 1985; Pyper et al., 1986; Yaniv et al., 1985). CAEV infection of goats elicits binding but not neutralizing antibodies. There is no evidence of selection of antigenic variants, however, variability in the virus genome during infection *in vivo* is still high.

Genetic structure and transcriptional control of lentiviruses

The organization and genetic content of the lentiviruses are very similar (Figure 1). Lentiviruses contain the same structural and enzymatic genes (*gag*, *env* and *pol*) as the retroviruses. In addition, there are small open reading frames that encode regulatory genes not found in other retroviruses. Visna virus has been studied in our laboratory and this review will focus on those studies, in particular, the role of the long terminal repeats (LTR) in the regulation of viral gene expression. The viral LTR contains the promoter/enhancer elements that interact with both cellular transcription factors and viral encoded transacting factors, that activate gene expression (Figure 2). The viral transacting factor, Tat, functions through the viral LTR to upregulate gene expression at both the transcriptional and post-transcriptional levels. The viral Tat protein acts on the promoters of cellular genes and upregulates cellular gene expression. This latter effect may be directly involved in the pathogenesis of the disease.

The 5′ LTR of all retroviruses (including lentiviruses) control transcription of all the viral RNAs (Figure 2). The U3 region of the LTR contains the binding sites for cellular and viral transcription factors and the TATA box. Cellular transcription factors regulate the basal level of viral RNA transcription that is accomplished by the cellular RNA polymerase II. In the case of the visna virus LTR, there are cellular factors that act both at the core enhancer sequence as well as binding upstream in the U3 region. Some of these factors are constitutively present in cells while others are induced during different stages of cellular differentiation and activation. The cellular factors that are constitutively present in the cell are required for basal transcription of lentiviral LTRs, but apparently are not sufficient to activate viral RNA transcription to levels required for productive virus replication. Transcription from the LTRs requires the binding of specific cellular factors that are either produced transiently or are modified during T cell or monocyte/macrophage activation and differentiation. In visna virus, we have observed that monocytes isolated from infected sheep do not express viral mRNA by *in situ* hybridization (Gendelman et al., 1986; Zink et al., 1990). However, the monocytes contain proviral DNA that is transcribed only when the monocytes matures into macrophages (Gabuzda et al., 1989; Shih et al., 1992). Another important element in viral gene expression is the viral transactivating gene *tat*, that acts through the core enhancer sequences (Gdovin & Clements, 1992).

Activation of viral transcription by cellular factors

In the visna virus system, we have been interested in the cellular basis of virus latency and activation. The tightly controlled regulation of viral gene expression in monocytes and macrophages clearly plays a central role in this process. In addition, we have been interested in identifying both viral and cellular factors that activate genes in the macrophage and the virus, that leading to the dysregulation of macrophage function and the lymphoproliferative disease caused by visna virus in sheep.

To understand viral activation we needed to have large numbers of monocytes that could be manipulated to mature into macrophages. It is difficult to do this in sheep macrophages because of the need for large numbers of purified cells. The human monocytic cell line, U937, was

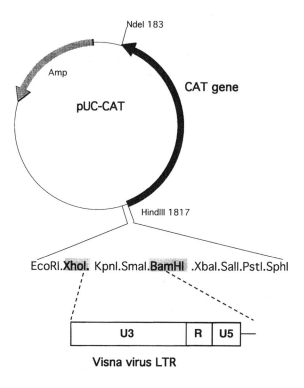

Figure 3a The visna virus LTR–CAT construct containing the U3, R and U5 sequences upstream of the bacterial CAT gene was constructed in the puc18 plasmid (Hess et al., 1989).

used in studies because they are monocytic cells that mature into macrophage when treated with phorbal esters (Rovera et al., 1979). The activity of the visna virus LTR was compared in the monocytic U937 cell, and the TPA-induced, U937 macrophage.

To examine the sequences responsible for transcriptional regulation, the visna virus LTR sequences (between −140 to +280) were placed upstream of the bacterial gene, chloramphenicol acetyltransferase (CAT) (Figure 3a). Activity from the promoter could be measured by transfection of the plasmid DNA into cells and enzymatic assay of the CAT protein produced in the cell (Hess et al., 1989). The differential expression of

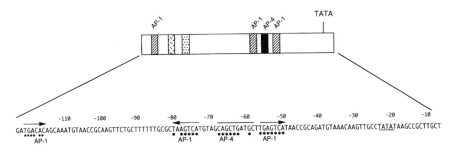

Figure 3b   The nucleotide sequence and location of binding sites for cellular transcription factors in the U3 region of the LTR. The boxes indicate the location of DNase I footprints in TPA treated U937 cells.

the visna virus promoter could be reproduced in the U937 cells. Low levels of CAT activity were measured in the U937 monocytes and the CAT activity was induced 4 fold in the TPA treated U937 macrophages. Quantitation of the CAT specific mRNA indicated that the increase in the steady state level of RNA accounted for the induced activity. Thus, this supported the idea that induction of gene expression was wholly at the transcriptional level (Gabuzda et al., 1989).

To identify the precise sequences in the promoter that were involved in this transcriptional activation, 5′ deletions (from −140 to −49) were made in the U3 sequences and were placed upstream of the CAT gene (Hess et al., 1989 (Figure 3b). When these deletion mutants were transfected into U937 cells and treated with TPA, it was found that the basal level of transcription decreased substantially when sequences were deleted to −111 (Gabuzda et al., 1989). However, there was still a difference in the level of CAT activity when the cells were treated with TPA in the −111, −91 and −81 deletion mutants. When sequences were deleted to −67, TPA inducible activity was lost. A similar result was obtained when the deletion mutants were transfected into primary human monocytes prior to treatment with TPA. Examination of the nucleotide sequences in this region of the viral promoter showed that the −67 mutant removed an AP−1 binding site and disrupted an AP−4 binding site (Angel et al., 1987; Bohmann et al., 1987; Mermod et al., 1988) (Figure 3b).

Cellular factors that activate transcription by interacting with AP–1 sites include members of the c–jun and c–fos family of oncogenes: these cellular factors are induced by TPA treatment of monocytic cells (Curran & Franza, 1988). Jun and Fos proteins form homo and heterodimeric complexes that activate transcription via AP–1 binding sites. The heterodimers of Jun and Fos bind DNA with a higher affinity than the Jun–Jun homodimers (Nakabeppu et al., 1988; Rauscher et al., 1988). AP–4 is another transcription factor induced by phorbol ester that activates transcription by acting in concert with AP–1 (Mermod et al., 1988).

To further investigate the role of cellular DNA binding proteins involved in the activation of the visna virus LTR in U937 monocytes and macrophages, nuclear extracts were generated at specific times after TPA treatment (Dignam et al., 1983). DNase I footprinting was done with these nuclear extracts of the LTR sequences from –140 to +22 revealed that there were three regions recognized by cellular proteins. Two of the regions showed identical DNase I protection patterns using nuclear extracts from either monocytic U937 cells or TPA-induced U937 cells.

In contrast to the constitutive binding, the region (–57 to –47) containing the AP–1 recognition site most proximal to the TATA box, showed inducible binding of cellular factors. There was only partial protection of this site with nuclear extracts from monocyte U937 cells, but the protection increased with the time of induction with TPA (Gabuzda et al., 1989). It has previously been demonstrated that multiple AP–1 binding sites are necessary to confer maximum TPA-inducibility on a promoter (Angel et al., 1987). We found that while all three AP–1 sites appear to be involved in the regulation of gene expression, the AP–1 site most proximal to the TATA box is clearly the most critical. In addition, this AP–1 site was DNase I-protected while the other two were not. Multiple binding sites for the same transcription factor are frequently of unequal importance, probably as a result of other variables such as proximity to the TATA box and flanking sequences.

It was now of interest to specifically identify the cellular proteins that bound to the visna virus promoter, specifically the region –49 to –59 that contained the AP–1 binding site. Since the cellular proteins Jun and Fos have been shown to bind to this sequence two approaches were used to show that these were indeed the cellular proteins involved in transcriptional activation of visna virus. To examine whether these cellular proteins bound to the AP–1 site in the visna virus LTR, a synthetic oligonucleotide containing the visna virus AP–1 sequence (–49 to –59) was used in gel-mobility shift assays with both TPA-induced U937 nuclear extracts and *in vitro* transcribed and translated Jun and Fos proteins (Shih et al., 1992). Gel shifts using the U937 nuclear extracts revealed the presence of a specific DNA-protein complex in TPA treated cells, whose intensity was greatest at 48 hours post-TPA-stimulation. The intensity of this complex was substantially reduced in extracts that had been pre-incubated with anti-Jun and anti-Fos antibodies, but were not reduced in the presence of an irrelevant antibody. Using *in vitro* synthesized proteins, Jun was found to bind to the visna virus AP–1 oligo, but as previously demonstrated, Fos alone did not bind to this sequence as it requires Jun for dimerization and DNA binding (Nakabeppu et al., 1988; Rauscher et al., 1988). An enhancement of binding was detected when both Jun and Fos were used for the binding studies (Nakabeppu et al., 1988; Rauscher et al., 1988). These results indicate that Jun and Fos are an integral part of the complex that binds and activates the visna virus LTR (Shih et al., 1992). It is also likely that other cellular components exist in this complex, as antibody interference assays did not completely inhibit binding to the visna virus AP–1 oligonucleotide.

In addition to protein binding, the level of the mRNAs of *c–jun* and *c–fos* were examined in the U937 cells. Little or no mRNA for either of these genes was present prior to TPA treatment, but it increased rapidly by 4 hours. The concentration of Jun and Fos proteins in the cells were also found to be increased with TPA treatment (Shih et al., 1992). Other studies have also shown that Fos mRNAs are upregulated by TPA treatment of U937 cells (Auwerx et al., 1990; Sherman et al., 1990). Thus, it appears that the cellular proteins Jun and Fos are important in the activation of viral gene expression in the monocytic cell line U937 and are likely to be involved *in vivo* in the activation of visna virus gene expression. This provides an example of how lentiviruses use host cell factors to activate expression of their viral genomes. It has been previously shown that the human immunodeficiency virus (HIV) uses the NF–kB and Sp–1 of factors to upregulate transcription from its LTR (reviewed in Jones, 1989).

Activation of viral transcription by the viral protein–tat

During the maturation of the macrophage, *c–jun* and *c–fos* are upregulated. As described above, these cellular proteins activate the visna viral LTR. The first proteins synthesized in the lentivirus life cycle are regulatory proteins; one of which is the transactivating protein, Tat. This protein increases viral transcription from the LTR via cellular transcription factors. The *tat* gene is encoded by the virus in a multiply spliced messenger RNA. The cDNA clone encoding the protein was used to study Tat protein function. The *tat* cDNA was transfected into vero cells along with a vector expressing the *neo* gene. A control cell line was transfected with only the *neo* gene. G418 was used to select Tat and *neo* expressing vero cells and *neo*-only expressing vero cells were used as a control cell line (Gdovin & Clements, 1992). Transfection of the viral LTR into the Tat cell resulted in 45 fold increase in activity over that observed in the control cell line. This increase in CAT activity was reflected at both the RNA and protein level (Gdovin & Clements, 1992).

To identify the target sequences in the viral LTR that responded to the visna Tat protein, a set of deletion mutants that begin at −140 and extend to −10 in the viral LTR were used (Hess et al., 1989). The LTR constructs were linked to the CAT reported gene and transfected into the Tat and control cell lines. These experiments showed that the AP–1 and AP–4 (−41 to −64) sites just upstream of the TATA box are the responsive sequences to Tat protein. It was found that other lentivirus LTRs that contain an AP–1 proximal to the TATA box were activated in the Tat cell line. These viruses include caprine arthritis encephalitis virus (CAEV), a closely related lentivirus, as well as feline immunodeficiency virus (FIV) (Table 2). The primate lentiviruses HIV–1 and SIV have AP–1 recognition sequences at the 5′ end of their U3 regions, yet these lentiviruses are not transactivated to any significant level by visna virus Tat (Table 2).

In addition, synthetic constructs were used to examine the role of the individual AP–1 and AP–4 sites in Tat transactivation. These constructs contained either one or two AP–1 sites or one AP–4 site (Table 3). Constructs containing either single or multiple AP–1 sites were activated by Tat. Activation, however, was at lower levels than the natural visna virus AP1/AP–4 sequence. The synthetic construct containing a mutated

Table 2.2. *Response of heterologous viral promoters to visna virus Tat*

Plasmid	Fold transactivation[c]
pVis LTR–CAT	46
pCAEV LTR–CAT	34
pFIV LTR–CAT	20
pHIV–1 LTR–CAT	9
pSIV LTR–CAT	8
pTK–CAT[d]	1.5

[c]Fold transaction was calculated by dividing levels of CAT activity in the Tat cell line by the levels in the control neo cell line.
[d]Herpes simplex thymidine kinase (TK) promoter.

AP–1 site (TGAGTCA-wild type; TTAGTCA-mutated) was not activated in the Tat cell line (Gdovin & Clements, 1992) (data not shown). This mutation in the AP–1 site has been shown to eliminate binding of the cellular proteins Jun and Fos (Nakabeppu et al., 1988). These data strongly suggest that the visna virus Tat protein acts through the AP–1 site.

Table 2.3. *Tat activation of visna virus LTR constructs and synthetic AP–1 & AP–4 constructs*

Plasmid[a]	Induction of CAT Activity[b]
pVIS–67 LTR–CAT	100
pVis–49 LTR–CAT	18
AP–1/–49 LTR–CAT	26
AP–1x2/–49 LTR–CAT	35
AP–4/–49 LTR–CAT	31

[a]pVIS–67 LTR–CAT contains the AP–1/AP–4 sites while pVis–49 LTR–CAT has no AP–1 or AP–4 sites. The AP–1, AP–1x2, and AP–4/–49 LTR CAT constructs have synthetic sites placed upstream of the pVis–49 LTR–CAT construct.
[b]Induction of CAT activity was calculated by dividing CAT activity in Tat cell lines by that in neo control cell lines, and is given as a percentage of the induction level for pVis–67 LTR–CAT.

However, no direct DNA–protein binding by Tat protein to this site could be detected in gel mobility shift assays. Thus, the Tat protein appears to act through the interaction with cellular proteins, most likely Jun and Fos.

The synthetic construct containing the AP–4 site was also found to be responsive to the Tat protein in the Tat cell line. However, like the synthetic AP–1 constructs the level of activation was about half that of the natural sequence in viral LTR (Table 3). The level of action of the Tat protein was examined for each of the synthetic constructs and there was an equivalent increase in RNA and protein suggesting that Tat acted at the transcriptional level. Nuclear run-on experiments further showed that the Tat protein acts at the level of transcription initiation (Gdovin & Clements, 1992).

Thus, visna virus gene expression is regulated both at the cellular and viral level via a core enhancer sequence that contains AP–1 and AP–4 binding sites. Cellular differentiation of the monocyte to the macrophage requires the upregulation of *c-jun* and *c-fos*. These transcription factors activate the visna viral LTR that controls gene expression. The viral Tat gene is one of the first viral proteins to be translated and functions to further activate viral transcription by interaction of cellular proteins at AP–1 sites.

Further, the Tat protein has been found to activate promoter elements both viral and cellular that contain AP–1 sequences. Thus, the function of the Tat protein in the virus life cycle may be both to increase viral gene expression and to activate cellular genes in the infected cell required for active viral transcription and replication. The *c–jun* and *c–fos* genes are rapidly upregulated as monocytes differentiate into macrophages but they are rapidly down regulated in the macrophage. There is only a transient expression (4–12 hours) of these transcription factors in the macrophage. The AP–1 site in the viral LTR is activated by these cellular factors and the down regulation of *c–jun* and *c–fos* would negatively affect virus gene expression. Thus, for active viral transcription Jun and Fos proteins are required in the cell. It has been found that the c–*fos* promoter is activated in the Tat containing vero cells (Gdovin & Clements, unpublished observations). In addition, *c–jun* expression is higher in visna virus infected cells (Neuvet et al., 1993). These data suggest that the Tat protein activates the expression of cellular transcription factors required for activated transcription from the viral LTR.

Conclusions

Visna virus infects monocytes and the viral genome is integrated into the cellular DNA. The provirus remains silent until the monocyte matures into a macrophage. Intrinsic to this maturation is the induction of a class of immediate early genes in the monocyte that includes the transcription factors Jun and Fos. These transcription factors are thought to couple short-term signals in the cell to long term cellular differentiation by regulation of specific cellular genes. Thus, Jun and Fos bind to the AP–1 site in the promoters of cellular genes and activate their transcription resulting in maturation of the monocytic to a macrophage. In addition, these cellular factors activate the same AP–1 sequence in the visna virus LTR leading to transcriptional activation, full viral gene expression and production of progeny virus. The expression of viral antigens in the infected macrophage results in antigen presentation in the context of MHC Class II. Infection of the macrophage also leads to the production of cytokines and a lymphoproliferative response that causes the lesions in specific target organs in an infected animal. We still only understand the framework of these events. The specific mechanisms by which viral genes alter macrophage gene expression and the molecular basis of visna viral tropism for specific tissue macrophages i.e. microglia still remains to be determined.

The possibility that the Tat protein activates cellular factors required for continued virus replication is intriguing. The activation of cellular genes that contain AP–1 sites may also be involved in the pathogenetic processes of the virus. The infected macrophage in target organs is responsible for the lymphoproliferative response causing clinical lesions. The cellular changes in the macrophage that lead to these responses may be due to the inappropriate activation of cellular genes by the Tat protein. The mechanism of action of visna Tat is being investigated as well as the identification of cellular genes that are affected by Tat expression. The Tat protein appears to be an important genetic element in viral gene expression and may play a key role in viral pathogenesis.

Acknowledgments

We thank Maryann Brooks for preparation of the manuscript. The studies reviewed were supported by grants from the NIH to Dr. J.E. Clements (NS23039 and AI07394).

References

Angel, P., M. Imagawa, R. Chiu, B. Stein, R. J. Imbra, H. J. Rahmsdorf,C. Jonat, P. Herrlich, and M. Karin (1987). Phorbol ester-inducible genes contain a common cis-element recognized by a TPA-modulated trans-acting factor. *Cell 49*:729–739.

Auwerx, J., B. Staels, and P. Sassone-Corsi (1990). Coupled and uncoupled induction of fos and jun transcription by different second messengers in cells of hematopoietic origin. *Nucl. Acids Res. 18*:221–228.

Bohmann, D., T. J. Bos, A. Admon, T. Nishimura, P. K. Vogt, and R. Tjian (1987). Human protooncogene c-jun encodes DNA binding protein with structural and functional properties of transcription factor AP-1. *Science 238*:1386–1392.

Chiu, I. M., A. Yaniv, J. E. Dahlberg, A. Gazit, S. F. Skuntz, S. R. Tronick, and S. A. Aaronson (1985). Nucleotide sequence evidence for relationship of AIDS retrovirus to lentiviruses. *Nature 317*:366–368.

Clements, J. E., S. L. Gdovin, R. C. Montelaro, and O. Narayan (1988). Antigenic variation in lentiviral dise. es. *Ann. Rev. Immunol. 6*:139–159.

Curran, T. and B. R. Fran a (1988). Fos and Jun: The AP-1 connection. *Cell 55*: 395–397.

Dignam, J. D., R. M. Lebowitz, and R. G. Roeder (1983). Accurate transcription initiation by RNA polymerase II in a soluble extract from isolated mammalian nuclei. *Nucl. Acids Res. 11*:1475–1489.

Gabuzda, D. H., J. L. Hess, J. A. Small, and J. E. Clements (1989). Regulation of the visna virus long terminal repeat in macrophages involves cellular factors that bind sequences containing AP-1 sites. *Mol. Cell. Biol. 9*:2728–2733.

Gdovin, S. L. and J. E. Clements (1992). Molecular mechanisms of visna virus tat: identification of the targets for transcriptional activation and evidence for a post-transcriptional effect. *Virology 188*:438–450.

Gendelman, H. E., O. Narayan, S. Kennedy-Stoskopf, P. G. E. Kennedy, Z. Ghotbi, J. E. Clements, J. Stanley, and G. Pezeshkpour (1986). Tropism of sheep lentiviruses for monocytes: Susceptibility to infection and virus gene expression increase during maturation of monocytes to macrophages. *J. Virol. 58*:67–74.

Hess, J. L., J. A. Small, and J. E. Clements (1989). Sequences in the visna virus long terminal repeat that control transcriptional activity and respond to viral trans-activation: involvement of AP-1 sites in basal activity and trans-activation. *J. Virol. 63*:3001–3015.

Jones, K. A. (1989). HIV trans-activation and transcription control mechanisms. *New Biol. 1*:127–135.

Mermod, N., T. J. Williams, and R. Tjian (1988). Enhancer binding factors AP-4 and AP-1 act in concert to activate SV40 late transcription *in vitro*. *Nature* 332:557–561.

Nakabeppu, Y., K. Ryder, and D. Nathans (1988). DNA binding activities of three murine JUN proteins: Stimulation by FOS. *Cell* 55:907–915.

Narayan, O. (1983). Role of macrophages in the immunopathogenesis of visna-maedi of sheep. *Prog. Brain Res.* 59:233–235.

Narayan, O., and J. E. Clements (1989). Biology and Pathogenesis of Lentiviruses. *J. Gen. Virol.* 70:1617–1639.

Narayan, O. and J. E. Clements (1990). Lentiviruses. In *Virology* ed. B. N. Fields & D. M. Knipe et al. New York: Raven Press Ltd. 2nd edition: 1571–1589.

Pyper, J. M., J. E. Clements, M. A. Gonda, and O. Narayan (1986). Sequence homology between cloned CAEV and visna virus, two neurotropic lentiviruses. *J. Virol.* 58:665–670.

Rauscher, F. J., P. J. Voulalas, B. R. Franza, and T. Curran (1988). FOS and JUN bind cooperatively to the AP-1 site: Reconstitution *in vitro*. *Genes Dev.* 2:1687–1699.

Roberson, S. M., T. C. McGuire, P. Klevjer-Anderson, J. R. Gorham, and W. P. Cheevers (1982). Caprine arthritis-encephalitis virus is distinct from visna and progressive pneumonia viruses as measured by genome sequence homology. *J. Virol.* 44:755–758.

Rovera, G., D. Santoli, and C. Damsky (1979). Human promyelocytic leukemia cells in culture differentiate into macrophage like cells when treated with a phorbol diester. *Proc. Nat. Acad. Sci.* 76:2779–2783.

Sherman, M. L., R. M. Stone, R. Datta, S. H. Bernstein, and D. W. Kufe (1990). Transcriptional and post-transcriptional regulation of c-jun expression during monocytic differentiation of human myeloid leukemic cells. *J. Biol. Chem.* 265:3320–3323.

Shih, D. S., L. M. Carruth, M. Anderson, and J. E. Clements (1992). Involvement of FOS and JUN in the activation of visna virus gene expression in macrophages through an AP-1 site in the viral LTR. *Virology* 190:84–91.

Yaniv, A., J. E. Dahlberg, S. R. Tronick, I. M. Chiu, and S. A. Aaronson (1985). Molecular cloning of integrated caprine arthritis-encephalitis virus. *Virology* 145:340–345.

Zink, M. C., J. A. Yager, and J. D. Myers (1990). Pathogenesis of lentiviruses: Cellular localization of viral transcripts in tissues of goats infected with caprine arthritis-encephalitis virus. *Am. J. Pathol.* 136:843–854.

3

Comparative epidemiology of human retroviruses

William Blattner, M.D.
Deputy Director
Institute of Human Virology
725 W. Lombard Street
Baltimore, MD 21201, USA

Introduction

The emergence of a worldwide epidemic of human immunodeficiency virus (HIV)-acquired immunodeficiency syndrome (AIDS) has stimulated an increased interest in human retroviruses. The discovery of HIV, a human retrovirus and the cause of AIDS, has its scientific lineage in the pioneering basic research done by Rous at the turn of the century inducing sarcomas in chickens,[208] the discovery of reverse transcriptase (RT) in the late 60s and early 70s[12,240] and the development of laboratory culture techniques using T-cell growth factors which made possible the isolation of the first human retrovirus, human T-lymphotropic virus type I (HTLV–I) by Gallo and his colleagues in 1979.[195] The isolation of HTLV–I established the existence of *human* retroviruses and laid the groundwork for detecting and growing other retroviruses such as HTLV–II, HIV–1 and HIV–2.[13,198]

Human retroviruses fall into three classes: oncornaviruses, lentiviruses and spumaviruses. HTLV–I and HTLV–II are classified as oncornaviruses; they occur in an endemic pattern, cluster geographically and are associated with a variety of clinical conditions including leukemia and degenerative neurologic disease. HIV–1 and HIV–2, the etiologic agents of AIDS, are lentiviruses with worldwide incidence. Antibodies to spumaviruses have been detected in some human populations but no disease association has been identified.[69] Until the discovery of HTLV–I in 1979, there was little confidence that a human retrovirus would be found because years of research had failed to find the expected viremic retrovirus in the pattern observed in experimental animal models. However, since neither HTLV–I nor HIV–1 maintain significant viremia, except during seroconversion (and in the case of HIV–1 at relatively low levels throughout the course of disease), the experimental animal models presented serious limitations. It was not until innovations in the culture of T-cells and in the detection of low level viral reverse transcriptase (RT) that the human retroviruses were discovered.

There are notable similarities between HTLV–I, HTLV–II and HIV based on shared functional activity of transactivating genes called *tax* for HTLV–I/II and *tat* for HIV–1/2, but they are distinctly different in how they interact with the host immune system and how they effect host cell growth.[74]

The HTLV and HIV viruses are single stranded RNA viruses containing a diploid genome which replicates through cDNA, a proviral intermediate[248] (Varmus, 1988). Reverse transcriptase, a viral enzyme, converts single stranded viral RNA into a double-stranded DNA provirus which is then integrated into the host genome by a viral integrase.[248] This genomic integration allows retroviruses to cause lifelong infection and diseases of long latency while evading immune clearance.[92,256]

Morphologically, HTLV–I is approximately 100 nm in diameter with a thin electron-dense outer envelope and an electron-dense, roughly spherical core. HIV–1 has a diameter of approximately 110 nm and is distinguished from the HTLV family by a cylindrical electron dense core (Figure 1: EM Photo). Retroviral genes generally code for large overlap-

---

Figure 1   Electron micrographs of HTLV–I and HIV1. In the upper panel for each virus is shown the budding particle; in the lower panel, the mature virion. (From Blattner, W. A.: Retroviruses. In Evans, A. S. (ed.): Viral Infections of Human Epidemiology and Control. 3rd edition. New York, Plenum, 1989, pp. 545–592.)

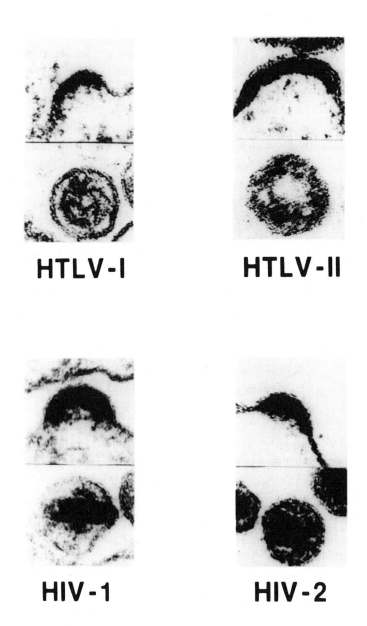

Figure 1

ping polyproteins that are later processed into functional peptide products by the viral encoded protease and cellular proteases.[248] Molecular sequencing of the HTLV and HIV viruses demonstrates the presence of long terminal repeats (LTR) at the 5' and 3' end of the genome which contain various regulatory elements.[76] The genomic structure 5' to 3' is similar for both viruses and contains the following genes: the *gag* (group-specific antigen), *pol* (polymerase/integrase), *env* (envelope), and a series of accessory genes which regulate virus expression.[73,74] The *gag* gene-related peptides for both viruses are synthesized from a single message and the peptides are formed through enzymatic cleavage employing the viral-encoded protease. The peptides function as structural proteins of the matrix, capsid and the nucleocapsid; the molecular weights are of similar size for both viruses. These peptides are strongly antigenic and appear as distinct bands in Western blots which are used to confirm the presence of antibody with molecular weights (MW) of 15,000 (p15), 19,000 (p19), 24,000 (p24), an intermediate breakdown product 28,000 (p28), and a precursor 53,000 (p53). The *pol* gene codes for several enzymes; reverse transcriptase (involved in RNA to DNA transcription), endonuclease (ribonuclease–H), and integrase which function for viral integration. The *env* gene encodes the major components of the viral coat: the surface glycoprotein of 46,000 MW (gp46) for HTLV–I and 120,000 MW (gp120) for HIV–1; the transmembrane component of 21,000 MW (gp21) for HTLV–I and 41,000 MW (gp41) for HIV–1; and the precursor, gp61/68 for HTLV–I and gp160 for HIV–1.

The regulatory region encodes for a series of peptides with similar functions in both viruses; the HTLV *tax* and HIV *tat* are responsible for enhanced transcription of viral and cellular gene products. The *tax* protein of HTLV–1 has been postulated to play a critical role in leukomogenesis.[18,176] *Rex* (regulator of expression of virion proteins for HTLV) and *rev* (regulator for HIV) modulate in a complex fashion the transport of virion components in the production of virus particles. HIV–1 employs additional regulatory genes in its life cycle and although the function of some of these accessory genes is not clear, both HIV–1 and HIV–2 include elements thought to be involved in infectivity, virus release, and syncytia formation (see Figure 2).

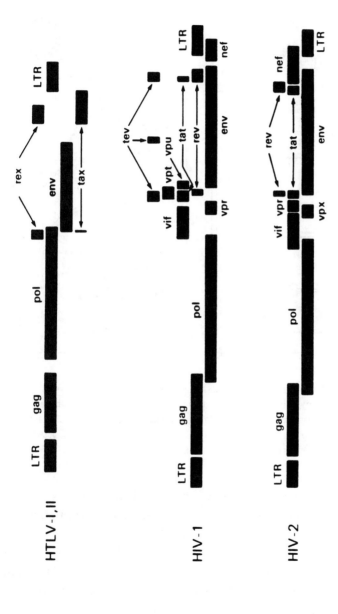

Figure 2 Retroviral Genomic Structures. The schematic depiction of the HTLV and HIV genomes shows that HTLV has a more complex genome than most animal retroviruses and HIV in turn has additional regulatory genes. The details of the function of each of these genes are summarized in the text. (From Gallo, R. C., Wong–Staal, F., Montagnier, L., et al.: HIV/HTLV gene nomenclature. Nature 333:504, 1988. Copyright 1988 Macmillan Magazines, Ltd.)

LIFE CYCLE OF HIV

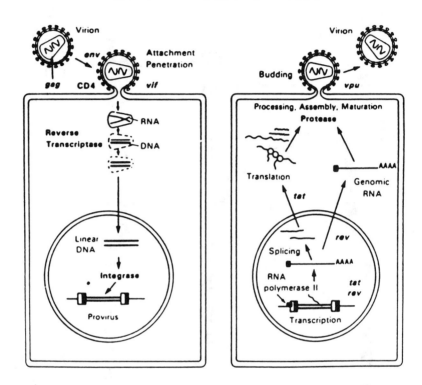

Figure 3   Life Cycle of HIV–1. In the left panel is shown the process of virus attachment and integration. In the right panel is shown the process whereby new infectious virions are produced. Details of these processes are discussed in the text. (from Gallo, R. C.: Mechanism of disease induction by HIV. J. AIDS 3:380–389, 1990. Copyright 1988 Macmillan Magazines Ltd.)

   The life cycle of the two classes of viruses is similar; it involves an infection phase (including viral attachment, entry, reverse transcription and proviral integration and an expression phase including transcription translation, assembly and budding of the virion)[248] (Figure 3). Both classes of virus attack the cells of the immune system. CD4 and CD8 are the major regulatory cells of the immune system; much of the pathogenesis that springs from these viruses is directly related to the critical role they play; when infected they cause immune dysfunction which seriously compromises the ability of the immune system to perform its myriad functions.

HTLV–I and HIV seem to be trophic for the CD4 positive lymphocyte[51] although it is clear that the CD4 molecule alone is not sufficient for virus binding of both viruses. The specific area for viral attachment of HTLV–I remains unknown although speculation has focused on a T-cell activation gene product on chromosome 17[230]. There continues to be considerable controversy concerning the nature of the second binding molecule for HIV–1; there is good evidence that HIV invades monocytes/macrophages;[178,197,199] experimental data shows that HTLV–I can also infect monocytes/macrophages. HTLV–II was isolated from a cell line that had CD4 positive cells but recent data suggests that the CD8 cell may be the major target for this virus.[111] Despite these differences, these viruses cause similar diseases: immunodeficiency, lymphoproliferative malignancies and neurologic syndromes. The median time from infection to disease for HTLV–I ranges from years to decades; for HIV–1 it may be 8–10 years or longer. In cases of HTLV–I-associated adult T-cell leukemia/lymphoma (ATL) the virus is monoclonally integrated in the cell but not at a specific site; recent data have raised the possibility that certain genomic sites may preferentially be chosen. In cases of HTLV–I-associated myelopathy (HAM/TSP) and other syndromes, integration is almost always polyclonal; less is known about HTLV–II integration but CD8 cells appear to be involved. Integration of HIV–1 appears to be random although a recent study reported non random integration of HIV–1 in juxtaposition to the c-*fos* oncogene in certain cases of non B–cell lymphoma in HIV–1 positive persons.[224]

There is wide variation in HIV–1 sequence around the world and over time in an individual; HIV transmission occurs through cell-free and cell-associated routes. This suggests that HIV–1 uses rapid genetic change as a means of evading immune surveillance and increasing efficiency of transmission. HTLV–I is remarkably constant from locale to locale (1 to 2% difference for most strains);[241] HTLV–I replicates at a much lower level and uses cell to cell transmission[75] which decreases the efficiency of transmission by an estimated order of magnitude less than HIV–1. HTLV–I tries to "hide" from the immune system[75,174,175] with a rate of change more consistent with "gene evolution." The most variant forms of HTLV–I differ by only 5–7% and these are found among isolates obtained from aboriginal peoples from Melanesia where the virus may have "evolved" in a population isolated from other sources of HTLV exposure.[81,258]

Viral origins

The question of where these viruses originated or how they got into humans is not known.[222,262] There is a long history of non-human primate to human transmission and a growing body of literature suggests that perhaps even HIV–1 can be sourced in this way.[121] The homology (primarily in old world primates) and among growing numbers of virus isolates from nonhuman primates (predominantly in Africa) show simian virus (SIVs) virtually indistinguishable from human viruses (HIV–2); this has prompted the proposal that these viruses be reclassified as "primate" retroviruses, PTLV and PIV.[17,77,221] The non human-to-human hypothesis is also supported by recent reports of some laboratory workers becoming infected with SIV and epidemiologic data presented in a study from Guinea-Bissau[77,123] where women involved in the preparation of primate meat for human consumption (with potential blood exposure) were at higher risk for HIV–2 infection. This might explain how this class of virus was introduced into humans who subsequently spread it through sexual and parenteral routes. It would also explain how such a highly sophisticated virus could appear in humans in such an explosive fashion promoted as it were through sociological and behavioral circumstances such as the breakdown of sexual taboos, coincident epidemics of sexually transmitted diseases, migration of populations from more rural to urban areas and drug abuse. Additional evidence is detected in new virus strains which diverge significantly from both HTLV–I and -II.[81,260] It is possible that additional examples of primate viruses and/or related human retroviruses will be discovered. Critical to this process is the ability to grow the target cell harboring the virus; recently developed molecular techniques for gene amplification may provide the additional tools needed for new virus detection.

Antigenic characteristics of HIV and HTLV

While HTLV–I and HIV–1 differ morphologically (see Figure 1) they share the structural features typical of human retroviruses (Figure 2). Several antigens of the core and envelope are strong immunogens and form the basis for a variety of serologic detection assays which employ whole viral and/or synthetic peptides in the detection of viral infection.[46,223,234] For the HTLV viruses the envelope antigens are immunogenic and are best detected in assays which employ synthetically produced peptides.[143] HTLV–I and HTLV–II are strongly cross reactive on standard screening assays; HTLV–II infections can be missed in the absence of either HTLV–II specific antigens or in assays "spiked" with recombinant p21 antigen[251] (Lal et al., unpublished data). The presence of antigen always signals the presence of virus infection as shown by a high concordance of culture and/or PCR positivity.[102,211] At the present time all studies indicate that infection is lifelong i.e. the virus is persistent producing infection for life although there are some instances of "abortive" infection detected by the presence of cell mediated immunity in the absence of culture and/or PCR proven infection. While state-of-the-art confirmatory tests use a variety of synthetic peptides to confirm virus type, previous studies used differential detection of p24 and p19 to distinguish HTLV–I from HTLV–II. HTLV–I has a strong reaction to both antigens; HTLV–II has a stronger p24 than p19 reaction. In most cases the absence of p19 and the presence of p24 is indicative of HTLV–II.[100,135,145,201] This algorithm has been used to evaluate virus type from large collections of sera obtained from different populations around the world. More recently, specific confirmatory antigens have been developed which facilitate typing; immunofluorescence assays are also used.

Epidemiology of HTLV–I/II

HTLV–I occurs in a worldwide distribution; the major foci occur in Japan, the West Indies, some areas of South America, Melanesia and in certain areas of Africa.[21] HTLV–II has been uncovered in the U.S. primarily among parenteral drug abusers and blood donors (about half of the blood donors are HTLV–II positive).[137,206,253] More recently clusters of HTLV–II infection have been found in native populations of North, Cen-

tral and South America; they vary by tribe and geographic locale.[91,97,106,140,151] HTLV–II is also found in some areas of West Africa
and, more recently, a pocket of PCR proven infection has been identified
in Mongolia among peoples who share certain genetic polymorphisms
with Amer-Indian peoples.[98]

Geographic distribution of HTLV–I/II

HTLV–I and –II are characterized by a pattern of endemic infection with
strong geographic clustering and evidence of persistent infection over decades.[21,93] The distribution of antibody positivity for both HTLV–I and
HTLV–II varies by geographic region and/or racial, ethnic and risk group
subpopulation.[21] HTLV–I clusters have been extensively reported in
southern Japan,[42,104] the Pacific Islands,[78,257,258] the Caribbean (primarily among immigrant descendants of the African slave trade),[23,29,41] some
countries in South and Central America[8,28,200,261] and in some locales of
sub-Saharan Africa.[54,83–85] Jewish migrants from the Mashad region of
Iran and Islamic peoples in the Mashad region of Iran.[161,225] The most
variant forms of the viruses occur among indigenous peoples in Melanesia, including Papua New Guinea,[81] Australia among aboriginal
peoples[16] and in some areas of Polynesia where the virus varies by as
much as 5 to 7% from the cosmopolitan strain of Japan, Africa and the
West Indies.[81,222,259]

HTLV–II infections cluster in the Americas, Africa and most recently
in Mongolia.[98] It is present in various Indian groups in South America but
not universally.[101,106,134,140,200] For example, HTLV–II is found in two
very isolated hunter gatherer tribes who share a common linguistic group
and reside on the Matogroso plateau in Brazil.[151] The very high rates of
HTLV–II infection here rival the very high rates reported for HTLV–I in
Okinawa.[119] Recent publications from several groups suggest an HTLV–
II-like virus in Africa[84] and among Mongolian people in Asia.[98] The
Mongolian virus closely resembles the one sequenced in the Americas;
the isolation and characterization of the African HTLV–II virus suggests
that it varies somewhat from the one isolated in the Americas.[97] Beyond
these locales, the worldwide distribution of HTLV–II is not fully characterized.[150]

Why the HTLV virus presents sporadically in these different endemic subpopulations is not clear. The differences between HTLV–I and HTLV–II may be plausibly explained by some prehistoric primate evolutionary break causing the viruses to evolve independently, first in non-human primates and later introduced through them into humans.[17] Other explanations include: they follow the migration patterns of some ancient peoples; the "founder effect" where small groups of infected individuals are responsible for infections in subsequent generations; and recently, the introduction of new routes of transmission i.e., parenteral drug abuse.[137]

Demographic patterns of HTLV–I/II

One of the characteristic features of HTLV–I is an age-dependent rise in seropositivity in viral endemic areas such as Jamaica, West Indies, Japan and others. This rise in seroprevalence becomes prominent in the adolescent years (Figure 4). The other characteristic feature of this age-dependent curve is the tendency for males to be less frequently infected than females. This is evident in Japan and in Jamaica regardless of the population under scrutiny; it reflects the relatively greater efficiency of transmission of HTLV–I from men to women than from women to men.[118,119,167] For HTLV–II there is also a striking age dependent rise in prevalence[151] but studies among the Guyami in Panama and the Kraho and Cayapo tribes from Brazil showed no differences in the rate of infection between males and females (Vitek, Blattner, et al., unpublished data). In this respect the pattern for HTLV–II more closely resembles the pattern seen for HIV–1 where there is more or less equal male to female ratio in heterosexual populations. The question of whether some of this age-dependent rise in HTLV prevalence could be the result of perinatal latent infection which does not express itself through the presence of antibody has been raised. Studies of one of the well-defined exposure groups such as seronegative children of seropositive mothers who have been breast-fed for extended periods of times (up to two years) have been undertaken. Nested PCR results document that none of the seronegative offspring of seropositive mothers who breast-fed their infants were positive as were the seropositive offspring who served as controls.[186,252]

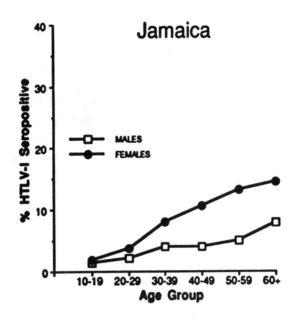

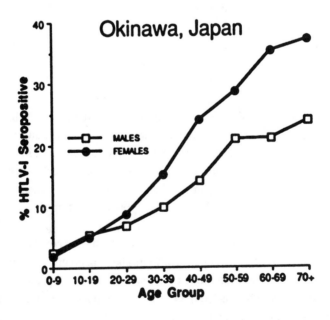

Modes of transmission

The modes of transmission for HTLV are from mother-to-infant, sexual intercourse and parenteral routes, i.e., intravenous drug use (IVDU) or transfusion (Table 1).

Transfusion and Parenteral

A patient transfused with a unit of HTLV–I-infected whole blood seroconverts about half of the time;[153,154,177,233] seroconversion is always associated with cellular products; plasma products do not transmit the HTLV virus because of its cell-association. In fact, HTLV–I-infected whole blood becomes less infectious as it is stored in the blood bank reflecting the gradual loss of infected lymphocytes from the blood unit.[154,177,233] Recipients of HIV–1 infected whole blood become positive 90% of the time.[58,59]

Sexual

Sexual transmission of retroviruses is more efficient from male to female although the converse does occur.[167] The cofactors for sexual transmission for HTLV–I and HIV–1 are complex. In prospective studies of HTLV–I discordant Japanese couples, older age and higher antibody titer were associated with transmission. Higher antibody titer appears to be reflective of HTLV–I virus load, a conclusion supported by semi-quantitative PCR which shows a correlation between virus load and antibody titer.[234] In studies of attenders of sexually transmitted disease clinics (STD) in the West Indies, a large number of partners and evidence of ul-

---

Figure 4   Seroprevalence of HTLV by age in Jamaica and Okinawa showing the similarity of the shape of the curve. (Jamaica: Reproduced with permission of Murphy E. L., Figueroa, J. P., Gibbs, W. N. et al. Human T-lymphotropic virus type I (HTLV–I) seroprevalence in Jamaica: I. Demographic determinants. Am. J. Epidemiol. 1991; 133:1114–1124. Okinawa: Kajiyama, W., Kashiwagi, S., Norura, H., Ikematsu, H., Hayashi, J., Ikematsu, W. Seroepidemiologic study of antibody to adult T-cell leukemia in Okinawa, Japan. Am. J. Epidemiol. 1985; 123:41–47.)

Table 3.1 *Transmission of HTLV–I*

HTLV–I: Modes of Transmission

Mother-to-Infant
  Transplacental
  Breast Milk
Sexual
  Male to Female
  Female to Male
  Male to Male
Parenteral
  Blood Transfusion
  Intravenous Drug Use

Cofactors

Elevated Virus Load
  Mother to Infant
  Heterosexual
Ulcerative Genital Lesions
Cellular Transfusion Products
Sharing of "injection works"

cerative genital disease, such as measured by VDRL status for syphilis, are documented transmission risk factors.[167] For HIV–1, lesions which disrupt the integrity of the genital mucosa facilitate transmission from female to male; coincident sexually transmitted disease in a female also heightens risk.[67]

Mother-to-child

Perinatal and transplacental HTLV–I mother-to-child transmission occur with 1–2% infection rates; the vast majority of the 20 to 25% of children are infected through breast feeding;[7,103,110,125,168] this contrasts with

Table 3.2   *HTLV–I associated diseases**

CHILDHOOD	
Infective Dermatitis	++++
Persistent Lymphadenopathy	++
Infant Death	+
Adult T-cell Leukemia/Lymphoma	+++
HTLV-Associated Myelopathy	++++
ADULT	
Adult T-cell Leukemia/Lymphoma	++++
Tropical Spastic paraparesis/ HTLV-Associated Myelopathy	++++
Infected Dermatitis	+++
Polymyositis	++
Uveitis	+++
HTLV-associated Arthritis	+++
Pulmonary Infiltrative Pneumonitis	++
Invasive Cervical Cancer	+
Small cell carcinoma of lung	+

*Key
++++   Proven association
  +++   Probable association
    ++   Likely association
      +   Possible association

HIV–1 where the infection rate is around 20% and the majority of the infections occur through perinatal exposure.

HTLV-associated diseases

The diseases associated with HTLV–I are listed in Table 2. One of the clinical manifestations of HTLV-associated diseases is adult T-cell leukemia (ATL), first described by Takatsuki in Japan[236–239,244] and subsequently confirmed in the Caribbean;[22,23,29] and a disease called Tropical Spastic Paraparesis/HTLV–I-Associated Myelopathy (TSP/HAM),[80] a chronic degenerative neurologic disease characterized by demyelination of the spinal cord and spastic paraparesis and polymyositis.[82,179,180] About a third of the cases of polymyositis in Jamaica are HTLV-associated.[166] Other HTLV-associated diseases include arthropathy, a large joint arthropathy described in Japan and uveitis of the eye.[164,171] Also being investigated are subtle hematologic abnormalities including anemia and skin test anergy.[235] There is some indication that persons with cancers in Japan are more likely to have HTLV antibodies, particularly invasive cervical cancer.[11,157] This may suggest a synergy between HTLV–I and invasive cervical cancer or it may be a reflection of their shared modes of transmission. A remarkable finding is that HTLV-infected individuals coinfected with HIV–1 progress more rapidly to clinical AIDS.[14]

Infective Dermatitis (ID) is an eczema-type skin disease characterized by chronic infections with saprophytic, staph and strep infections; these can be treated with antibiotics but recur if the antibiotic regimen is stopped.[132] The original cases of infants and children described in the late 60s and early 70s have been followed and the illness persists in these now young and middle-aged adults.[99] Some have gone on to develop adult T-cell leukemia; others have developed the neurologic syndrome.[133] It is now postulated that this syndrome is effected through perinatal HTLV infection of an immature immune system although some recent cases have been ascribed to adult HTLV–I exposure. The attack on the immune system of the susceptible host results in a rather targeted and subtle form of immune deficiency which in turn causes infective dermatitis. In addition to infective dermatitis, other identified childhood manifestations include pediatric versions of TSP/HAM and adult T-cell leukemia. Some data also raise the possibility that rates of infant death among children born to HTLV positive mothers are elevated,[252] but this finding could be confounded by lower socioeconomic class. Other evidences of HTLV as an immunosuppressive virus include the frequent association of HTLV infection with refractory and clinically disseminated strongyloidiasis and Norwegian scabies and AIDS-like illnesses in the absence of HIV.

HTLV–II-associated diseases are still undetermined (Table 3). There are case reports suggesting the possibility of HTLV–II disease-associa-

Table 3.3 *Suspect HTLV–II associated diseases**

	CHILDHOOD
Glomerular Nephritis	+

	ADULT
T-Hairy cell/Large Granulocytic Leukemia	++
HTLV-Associated Myelopathy/ Tropical Spastic Paraparesis	++
Eczema	+
HTLV-associated Arthritis	+/–
Asthma	+

*Key
++ Likely association
+ Possible association
+/– Weak association

tion but none have been confirmed. HTLV–II was originally isolated from a patient diagnosed with atypical T-cell hairy cell leukemia;[120] a second case was subsequently reported in a patient with hairy cell leukemia of B–cells[205] and in a few recent cases large granulocytic leukemia has been reported in association with HTLV–II.[97,147,155] And, while it is possible that all of these cases represent variants of the same disease entity to date no consistent pattern has been observed. There are reported individual cases of HTLV–II-associated neurologic disease resembling TSP/HAM and its variants made in the context of blood transfusion in the U.S. and Panama.[92,105,114] However in both studies, the frequency of HTLV–II-associated disease was less frequent than in cases associated with HTLV–I. This may indicate that both viruses cause a TSP/HAM-like illness but more frequently in association with HTLV–I. Other studies being done in Panama raise the possibility of a link to asthma in adulthood; several other case studies have also raised this possibility.

HTLV pathogenesis

The process of HTLV pathogenesis is not fully understood. The normal immune system responds to foreign agents such as viruses with a proliferation of T and B lymphocytes.[115,128] One effect of the HTLV virus on the immune system is spontaneous lymphocyte proliferation, polyclonal expansion, and monoclonal expansion resulting in a malignant phenotype (Figure 5). If lymphocytes from HTLV carriers are put in a test tube the level of cell proliferation rivals those which result when a mitogen-like PHA is put into the test tube—there is a spontaneous lymphocyte proliferation. Other antigens in tropical environments also may enhance spontaneous lymphocyte proliferation in noninfected cells. This would increase targets by activating lymphocytes and thus allow HTLV to more easily infect the host. This initiates a cycle of lymphocyte proliferation which increase the numbers of infected cells and with it increased infectivity. Most importantly, in terms of pathogenesis, polyclonal and monoclonal HTLV expansions can proceed in a number of ways: lymphoproliferation resulting in adult T-cell leukemia; immune dysregulation resulting in a panoply of autoimmune-like disease that seem to be HTLV-associated (Figure 5). HTLV–I seems to be both immunosuppressive *and* immunoproliferative and employs a different and perhaps more subtle but equally complex strategy for inducing disease than does HIV–1.

HIV

Epidemiology of HIV

The Centers for Disease Control and Prevention first described the epidemic now known as AIDS as an unexplained cluster of immunodeficient gay men residing in Los Angeles. This June 1981 report marks the beginning of what has become a worldwide pandemic whose death toll in the United States alone exceeds a quarter of a million persons. Worldwide, human losses are calculated in the millions; these numbers do not include those who are *not* counted, (especially in the developing countries) because of inadequate surveillance.[30]

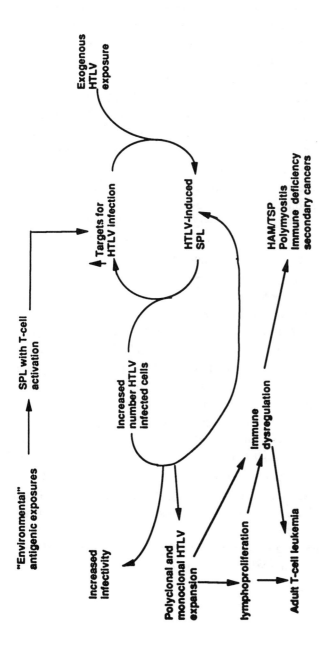

Figure 5 Interaction of HTLV and spontaneous proliferation of lymphocytes (SPL). Hypothesis of how immune activation as measured by spontaneous proliferation of lymphocytes might amplify risk of HTLV–I infection and thus explain some aspects of the peculiar geographic distribution of HTLV–I. This ongoing property of HTLV–I induced proliferation may contribute to the pathogenesis of both the leukemia and the neurologic and related conditions. (Prepared by W. A. Blattner and S. Wiktor from unpublished data.)

There are two distinct types of HIV: HIV–1 the etiologic agent responsible for the worldwide pandemic of AIDS and HIV–2 which is sometimes associated with AIDS but appears to be less virulent;[62,126] HIV–2
clusters primarily in West Africa.

The origin of HIV in humans is unknown but it is now clear that the
HIV–1 epidemic began years before the first cluster of cases was identified.[36] The first documented HIV infection was seen in a British seaman
who died of progressive immunodeficiency in 1959.[45] Anecdotal cases
from the United States and Europe and the significant number of HIV
seropositives from Africa in the 1960s and 70s support the notion that the
virus has been present in humans for some years. New evidence increasingly supports the concept that the virus, with its highly adapted receptor
for the CD–4 molecule and its intricate array of viral regulatory proteins
for subverting cellular functions, is not new but rather a highly evolved
virus that has been newly introduced into man from an advanced sophisticated primate source (see page 58). Support for the enzootic origin of
HIV come from the recent discovery of an HIV–2 isolate from Liberia
that is virtually identical to an SIV strain.[77]

The pandemic HIV–1 contrasts markedly with endemic HTLV. As indicated earlier, HTLV–I and –II are geographically focused and have a
limited distribution; HIV–1 occurs throughout the world infecting large
numbers of persons via sexual and parenteral routes. HTLV–I displays
patterns of occurrence which appear to correspond with documented population migrations i.e., from Africa to the Americas as part of the slave
trade, or from Mongolia to the Americas as part of ancient migrations
across the Bering Straits; HIV–1 spread around the world reflects fundamental changes in modern societies, their behaviors, their migrations and
the global economy, not only in traditional goods and services, but also in
illicit drugs and commercial sex.[1] And, unlike HTLV–I and –II, the age
distribution tends to concentrate in the sexually active age group and in
the pediatric group, an epidemic pattern reflecting the behaviors of those
at risk and their offspring.[191]

Geographic distribution of HIV/AIDS

Testing historic collections of sera obtained before the HIV/AIDS era verify the worldwide introduction of HIV into various high risk populations and rapid increases in prevalence among different high-risk populations in the U.S., Europe and in Africa. By the early 1980s, the ways in which the HIV virus could be transmitted were known and this information was widely distributed. Unfortunately, the dissemination of this information did not change the pattern of new waves of infection as the epidemic expanded explosively throughout the U.S., Europe, and Africa[5,117] and recently on a grand scale in Southeast Asia and India (Figure 6).[172,181,209]

Through July 1993, 600,000 AIDS cases out of an estimated total worldwide of 2,500,000 were reported to the World Health Organization (WHO). Sixty-eight percent of this estimated worldwide total (1.8 million cases) occurs in the sub-Saharan countries of Africa; 10 to 15% in the United States; 14–15% in Europe and a small number in Asia and the Middle East (while the present number of AIDS cases in Southeast Asia are small i.e., 2.5% of the cases and 13% of the total HIV infections, signs of an impending epidemic are surfacing).[1] Among the countries with the highest total case load rate per 100,000 are the United States, 19.6; Uganda, 22.3; Malawi, 51.6; Kenya 24.7; Côte d'Ivoire, 28.3; and Tanzania, 15.5.[152] A number of studies have suggested that these figures seriously underestimate the problem. For example, even though 68% of the cases occur in sub-Saharan countries they report approximately 10–15% of the global total and, a recent survey in the capitol of Côte d'Ivoire confirmed HIV–1 was associated with over a third of all deaths (based on postmortem blood samples) and was similar to the United States as a leading cause of death for persons in the sexually active age group.[53] The Côte d'Ivoire survey is one example of how the lack of adequate medical services and the complexity of diagnosing AIDS and its protean manifestations can result in significant underestimation of the numbers of AIDS-infected people in the world. While projections for the total number of AIDS cases through the end of the 20th century vary widely, the Global AIDS Policy Coalition is projecting 15 million cases including 3 million women and children.[1]

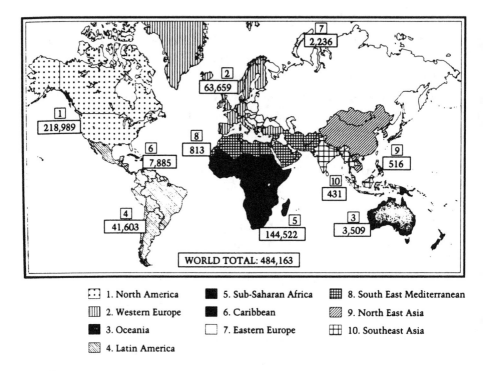

Figure 6   Emergent World Epidemics. The cumulative number of reported adult AIDS cases worldwide by Geographic Area of Affinity, through January 1, 1992. (Source: World Health Organization, Geneva, Switzerland, 1992. Reported as of April 3, 1992.)

Surveillance for AIDS, the endstage of HIV–1 infection, has been a more useful public health tool in developed countries with state-of-the-art medical care than in developing countries where the unavailability of health services places serious limits on diagnostic services.[86] Even with AIDS surveillance, the long latency period from infection to disease places limitations on the ability to accurately determine the current status of HIV infection and the dynamics of how it is spreading. Thus, HIV surveillance was a more useful tool in the detection of the emerging epidemic in Southeast Asia where large numbers of infections have occurred rapidly in a short period of time.[172,181]

In economically developed countries AIDS surveillance continues to be the cornerstone for understanding the magnitude of the epidemic, and for discerning trends and pattern shifts. An important use of AIDS surveillance data has been the application of statistical modeling techniques such as backcalculation for estimating the number of HIV infected persons.[202] Based on these data estimates in the range of 600,000 to 1 million persons have been estimated for the United States.

Demographic patterns of HIV/AIDS

Data concerning the underlying epidemic of HIV infection are critical to understanding the future course of the AIDS epidemic and to effecting strategies to stem the tide. Of the 9 to 15 million persons infected worldwide, over 1 million are children. In North America it is estimated that approximately 1 million persons are infected; this represents 1 in 75 males and 1 in 700 females between the ages of 15 and 49 years. In Latin America with an estimated 1 million infected, and Western Europe with 730,000 infected there is a similar male predominance in infection reflecting the impact of male homosexual and parenteral drug abuse exposure. In sub-Saharan Africa the male to female ratio is unity and approximately 1 in 30 males and females between 15 and 49 are HIV–1 infected. Overall 7.8 million persons in this region are estimated to be infected, including 969,000 infants and children.[1] In the countries of equatorial Africa including Zaire, Zambia, Rwanda, Kenya and Uganda and in West Africa in Côte d'Ivoire, infection rates of 5 to 10 percent are reported especially among general urban populations in the sexually active age group. Significant HIV infection is occurring in non urban populations as well and mathematical projections raise the possibility that, over the next decade, 15% to 20% of the work force in some areas of Africa may die; attendant social fallout will include up to 10 million orphans.[6] Asia and Southeast Asia represent areas where HIV is newly introduced but rapidly spreading. Already 675,000 persons are estimated to be infected mainly in India and Thailand with drug abuse and heterosexual transmission accounting for the rapid spread.

Serologic surveys in the United States primarily of military recruits, newborn infants and Job Corps applicants, provide a window to the status of the HIV epidemic and record seroprevalence trends over time. Among military recruits the highest rates of HIV-1 infection occur in the North-east and Mid-Atlantic region which tend to have a high rate for AIDS as well.[27] Crude seroprevalence for recruits is 1.42 per 1000 for men and 0.66 per 1000 for women. Peak occurrence is in the 25 to 30 year old age group; rates are higher in minority populations (4 per 1000 black male and 2.2 per 1000 hispanic males) compared to 0.5 per 1000 for whites. The rates of infection over time have declined from 1.5 per thousand in 1985 to less than 1 per 1000 currently; this reflects in part, the self exclusion of persons with lifestyles characteristically associated with high risk for HIV (e.g., drug abuse, gay sexual orientation) who are discouraged from participation in military service. Trends for both whites and blacks are similar; prevalence in whites declined from 1 per 1000 in 1985 to 0.5 per 1000 in 1989 and in blacks from 4 per 1000 to 2.7 per 1000 in the same time period. Job Corps applicants manifest trends similar to those observed for military recruits geographically and by race[32] rates range from 5.5 per 1000 for black males to 1.5 per 1000 for white males. However, female and male rates are more similar in Job Corps applicants than in military recruits. Trends in overall prevalence among blood donors have also shown a decline from 0.25 per 1000 in 1985 to less than 0.1 per 1000 currently. First time male blood donors' rate approached 0.9 per 1000 in 1985 and had stabilized at approximately 0.4 per 1000 by 1989. These trends most likely represent the positive impact of donor deferral programs and the exclusion of seropositives from future blood donation.[32]

All of these surveys, including hospital based surveys, are biased in various ways and work to either overestimate or underestimate the underlying seroprevalence in the community at large. However, these data support the conclusion that approximately 1 million persons in the United States are seropositive and that the epidemic is increasingly focusing on minorities and women.[216] The worldwide trend is moving toward spiralling infections among disadvantaged populations.[79,136]

Population surveyed and backcalculation

The variety of techniques used to monitor trends in HIV–1 incidence over time include retrospective surveys, prospective surveys, serial cross-sectional surveys and statistical techniques such as backcalculation.

Patterns of HIV–1 incidence among various risk groups are determined by using the backcalculation technique. Rates peaked in the early 1980s among gay men and recipients of blood products but continue to rise in intravenous drug using populations and high risk heterosexual groups.[26] The reasons given for the dramatic declines in HIV–1 incidence are the positive effects of safe sex campaigns and saturation of the pool of susceptibles could also explain these patterns.

Recent prospective surveys of sexually active gay men document disturbing patterns of high risk behavior and seroconversions in some young gay men, despite intensive educational efforts.[212,246] Intravenous drug users and their female partners are another groups previously cited with high rates of new infection.[56]

Rates of infection in broader segments of the population have been monitored by serial cross-sectional surveys of populations such as successive cohorts of military recruits and cohorts of active duty personnel who are repeatedly tested over time. For example, by utilizing annual data from military recruits, annual infection rates were estimated to be 0.14% for black men, 0.017% for white men, 0.052% for hispanics and 0.003% for white females.[27]

While the rates of new infection in the United States appear stable, the latest research documents increasing rates in many developing countries of the world, particularly in Africa, the Caribbean, South America, and Southeast Asia. Dramatic increases have been reported among Bangkok intravenous drug abusers and female prostitutes in Northern Thailand and in India.[156,169,213,227–229,245,247] Rising rates of HIV–1 have been observed among populations in sexually transmitted diseases clinics (STDs). Population based studies in some African countries document expanding epidemics among subsets of the general population including rural populations in Uganda and Tanzania.[124,250] Cohort studies of prostitutes in Nairobi, Kenya and Lagos, Nigeria have documented dramatic increases.[50,191]

In the future, a major focus of epidemiologic research must provide a more precise understanding of populations at greatest risk[25] and the dynamics of new seroconversions so that prevention campaigns and vaccine programs, when they become available, can be implemented to blunt the occurrence of new infections.

Modes of transmission

HIV–1 is transmitted by behaviors and circumstances which promote intimate exposure to infectious blood or bodily fluids containing the HIV virus and/or HIV infected cells. Blood and blood products (including plasma and derivatives), semen, vaginal secretions, breast milk, exudates but not transudates, and sometimes saliva are documented sources for exposure.[87] Gamma globulin and other highly processed and inactivated blood products are not infectious but HIV antibodies are detectable in these materials.[255]

Sexual

Sexual transmission is the major mode of HIV spread worldwide; heterosexual exposure accounts for approximately 75% of the 13 million infections worldwide[1] and male homosexual sex accounts for over half of the AIDS cases in the United States and other developed countries.[94] Recently, in the United States, heterosexual exposure and intravenous drug use—the sharing of unsterilized needles—have emerged as the major source of new infections among some, particularly inner city and minority populations.[109] In some developing countries, particularly in some areas of Africa and Eastern Europe, parenteral exposure to inadequately sterilized injection equipment has resulted in epidemics of nosocomial transmission.[210]

Transfusion and parenteral

Prior to the development of a blood screening assay, transfusion of HIV–1 infected blood and blood factor concentrates contributed to a significant number of infections.[58,59,130] The current generation of blood screening assays has made blood transfusion virtually risk-free. These new assays are highly sensitive and specific and have significantly narrowed the window for detecting infection during the shift from plasma viremia to antibody development. The increasing variability of the virus worldwide presents a challenge to current blood screening technologies and some risk persists in areas where new infections are occurring in large numbers and new variants appear. Recently a major HIV–1 variant was discovered in Equatorial Africa[158] which was missed by the current generation screening tests. An estimate derived from statistical modeling estimates that 1 in 225,000 blood units in the U.S. is potentially contaminated due to false negatives (e.g., recently infected antigen positive, antibody negative persons) or as a result of laboratory error. Laboratory error accounts for the bulk of the risk. Health care and laboratory workers are at increased risk when exposed to HIV–1 through needle stick or occasionally as a result of cutaneous or mucous membrane exposure to contaminated blood or bodily fluids.[37] The risk to a health care worker who experiences a single needle stick from an infected patient is approximately the same risk as a single unprotected sexual encounter without other contributing cofactors such as coincident STDs. Nonetheless, the laboratory workers can control their own risks for HIV transmission in the laboratory by observing "safety first" precautions.

Mother-to-infant

Mother-to-infant transmission is increasingly a problem around the world as the number of infected women increases.[20] The majority of infections occur via perinatal and/or perinatal exposure although breast feeding is also a means of infection in those areas of the developing world where non breast feeding is contraindicated because of high infant mortality due to diarrhea and other conditions. The rates of transmission range from approximately 10% to almost 50% depending on a number of factors including breast feeding and the immune status of the mother.[95,232] In developed countries the rate is approximately 15% with over half of this risk due to perinatal exposure in the birth canal; breast feeding is felt to contribute an additional 15% to the overall risk. In one Russian study, mothers were infected from saliva of their infants who had acquired HIV infection through transfusion; cracked or bleeding nipples served as a co-factor.[196]

Cofactors

Cofactors which contribute to heighten transmission include heterosexual or homosexual contact with multiple partners or sexual contact with a person with multiple partners or with a drug abusing partner.[116] Female commercial sex workers are at high risk for acquiring infection and spreading it to their clients.[129] Traumatic sexual contact such as anal intercourse or "fisting" or vaginal/penile abrasion are also linked to increased risk.[67] Other coincidental sexually transmitted diseases, especially ulcerative genital lesions, increase transmission risk even when controlling for the effect of multiple sexual partners.[226] Lack of male circumcision also heightens risk.[226] Intravenous drug users who share needles and injection equipment particularly in the context of multiple injection partners have a very high risk of transmission. Intravenous drug users in the mid-Atlantic and northeastern regions of the United States, including New York City and northern New Jersey have much higher rates than locales in the mid- or far West.[55] Worldwide, HIV–1 continues to spread through intravenous drug use and sexual transmission; the dramatic epidemic of HIV–1 in Thailand since 1987 is the result of both types of exposure.[156,229,247] Crack cocaine abuse also contributes to HIV–1 spread largely by increasing sexual transmission due to the proactive practice of bartering sex for drugs. Viral cofactors have also been suggested. Certain strains of virus may be more infectious because of their growth characteristics or cell trophism; this is exemplified in northern Thailand where the strain of virus is largely associated with sexual transmission while a different strain in Bangkok seems to be associated with the epidemic of drug-abuse associated infection.[40,181]

Other mediators in transmission

Virus load of the infectious partner (high virus titer being associated with increased likelihood of transmission) is a major determinant especially those with antigenemia or those with advanced immune compromises.[88,107] Immune response also influences transmission; findings in studies of mother-to-infant transmission suggest that rare "escape" mutants may evade immune surveillance.[254] Patterns of immune response to the envelope antigen of HIV–1 may influence transmission as well.[90,207,254] Host genetic characteristics may also influence the likelihood of transmission; there are well documented instances of highly exposed individuals who have not become infected. In a study of highly exposed Kenyan prostitutes some remained seronegative despite massive exposure; evidence of cell mediated immunity was found which might indicate an effective response to exposure to the virus.[194] It is possible that this response is genetically determined since certain rare alleles of the major histocompatibility complex were more frequent in those who were uninfected. Thus host determinants of immune response to virus exposure may allow for effective clearance of infectious virus.

Transmission probabilities

While the likelihood of transmission of HIV–1 varies by exposure route and various cofactors, the virus is generally poorly transmitted. For example, the probability of transmission from a single anal receptive sexual contact with an infected partner is estimated at 1 in 100 to 1 in 500; a single male to female vaginal sex act is estimated to result in transmission 1 in 500 to 1 in 1000 times while female to male transmission is thought to occur 1 in 1000 to 1 in 1500 times.[182] A single needle stick is thought to transmit the virus 1 in 400 to 1000 times.[31] The likelihood of a mother transmitting the virus to her infant is between 1 in 3 and 1 in 7 times.[90] Certain cofactors such as coincident sexually transmitted diseases, and high levels of circulating free virus appear to substantially augment transmission and might change the odds of a particular exposure resulting in an infection by as much as an order of magnitude. Interventions such as using condoms and sterile needles may reduce risk substantially.[3,4,38,144]

Women, children and HIV/AIDS

A recent trend worldwide is the emergence of AIDS in women and children; this trend has occurred concomitantly with the increasing spread of

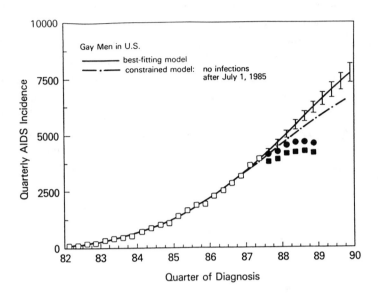

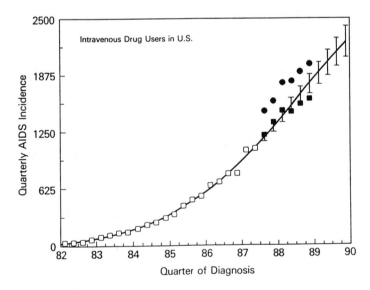

Figure 7

the virus through drug abuse or heterosexual transmission.[63,70] In some countries half of the AIDS cases are women; this upward trend has been tabulated in the United States for the last five years where women and children account for approximately 15 percent of all cases.[39]

Time trends in AIDS incidence

Time trends among risk groups provide interesting insights into the directions taken by the AIDS epidemic in the United States. Figure 7 shows that beginning in the second quarter of 1987 the incidence of AIDS among U.S. gay men began to level off declining to 55% of all the US cases from an earlier high of 70%; this pattern is not observed among intravenous drug abusers.[33] While it was hypothesized that this trend could have resulted from the positive benefits of behavior change in the homosexual population, this would not be only reason for such an abrupt decline. The most plausible explanation would be the improvement in therapy and prophylaxis, particularly the introduction of antiretroviral therapies such as Zidovudine, first introduced in the second quarter of 1987. The reasons for differences in rates among homosexual men versus intravenous drug users may relate to the greater access to care in the gay population.[72,203] Other data from various cohorts and treatment groups have documented the positive impact of therapy.

While antiretroviral therapy is having a positive impact on AIDS occurrence by delaying the progression of HIV positive individuals to AIDS, it is likely that this trend will reverse itself with the emergence of resistant strains.[2] There is considerable uncertainty regarding the long term effects of therapy since combinations of agents and the development of new therapies may continue to influence AIDS natural history. Furthermore, prolonged survival among HIV-1 positive individuals with severely depressed immunity may be associated with other adverse

---

Figure 7   AIDS incidence in the US over time. A) Gay men in the U.S. Solid line, unconstrained model. Dashed line, constrained model, i.e. no new infections since 1985. All cases observed (●). Cases consistent with pre-1987 cases (■). Intravenous drug users in U.S. Reproduced with permission from reference 67.

effects.[35,192,214] There is documented high incidence of non Hodgkin's lymphoma among a cohort of individual with less than 50 per mm^3 CD4 cells who experienced long term survival on antiretroviral therapy.[193] During a period of several years over 30% of these individuals developed lymphoma. Based on these data as well as trends in lymphoma surveillance, it is possible that 20% to 30% of all lymphomas among the at-risk age group in the 1990s may be HIV-associated.[71] Other long term sequelae such as HIV-associated neurologic disease and other chronic degenerative diseases not yet recognized will undoubtedly surface.[68,139]

Thus while therapy has a clear positive benefit, there are continued challenges, particularly the need to develop a variety of approaches which suppress the virus and thereby enhance the body's ability to clear out the virus and reconstitute the immune system. Nonetheless, a challenge that can be met today is to insure that all persons, regardless of socioeconomic status have access to the available, effective life-giving therapies. The disadvantaged in the United States and the million worldwide already infected with the virus should have access to these life-supporting therapies. AIDS has had a significant impact on death rates. Figure 8 clearly illustrates that over the last ten years, HIV/AIDS has emerged as the leading cause of death among U.S. men between the ages of 25–44 years of age; it now exceeds accidental injuries.[34] The social and economic ramifications represented by such a serious loss of human potential in the most productive age group is incalculable.

Natural history of HIV

The documented cause of AIDS is HIV–1. Some scientists and others have expressed doubts that HIV–1 causes AIDS and is responsible for the current pandemic because of the lack of understanding of the mechanism(s) by which the virus causes immune destruction. Figure 9 illustrates the hallmark in the natural history of AIDS which is the progressive decline in CD–4 lymphocytes over time.[108,185,188,215] The discovery of HIV–1 in 1983 and its continuous production in 1984 provided *in vitro* evidence that the putative cause was CD–4 trophic and caused destruction of T-lymphocytes, a pattern which mimicked the progressive destruction of immunocytes *in vivo*.[57,74] Prospective and cross sectional epidemio-

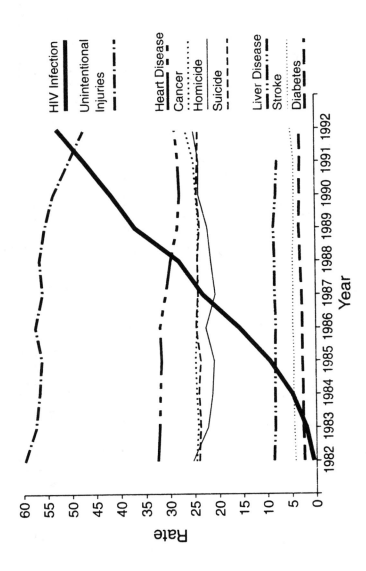

Figure 8   CDC leading causes of death among men aged 25–44 years, by year—United States, 1982–1992. Per 100,000 population. National vital statistics based on underlying causes of deaths, using final data for 1982–1991 and provisional data for 1992. Data for liver disease in 1992 are unavailable. CDC. MMWR Morbidity and Mortality Weekly Report 1993; 42(45):871

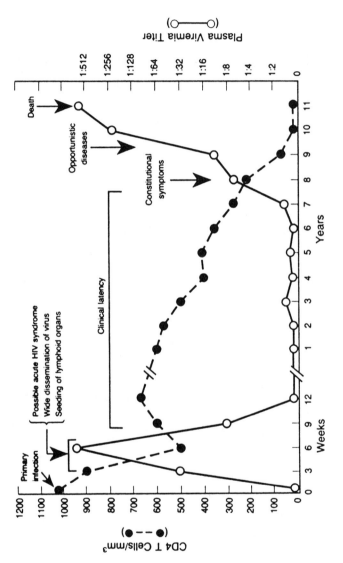

Figure 9   Typical course of HIV infection (virus load and CD4 T-cell decline). During the early period after primary infection there is widespread dissemination of virus and a sharp decrease in the number of Cd 4 T-cells in peripheral blood. An immune response to HIV ensues with a decrease in detectable viremia followed by a prolonged period of clinical latency. The CD4 T-cell count continues to decrease during the following years until it reaches a critical level below which there is a substantial risk of opportunistic diseases. Pantaleo, G., Graziosi, C., Demarest, J. F., et al., HIV infection is active and progressive in lymphoid tissue during the clinically latent stage or disease. Nature 1993; 362: 355–358.

logic studies convincingly linked HIV as the etiologic cause of AIDS by showing that HIV–1 was an exposure necessary to the subsequent occurrence of AIDS. However, a lack of full understanding of the pathogenic process has limited understanding of exactly *how* the virus causes AIDS. The development of more sophisticated molecular probes and approaches has provided new insights elucidating the process from seroconversion to end stage failure of the immune system.[66,190] The initial target of infection is either the dendritic,[61] the CD4 lymphocyte and/or the monocyte–macrophage—probably depending on the mode of exposure and the trophism of the virus. Nothing is known about the subsequent trafficking of the virus until a detectable burst of viremia some weeks following initial exposure.[49,148] This initial viremia is cleared by an immunologic host response with substantial reduction in virus load *and* a concomitant reduction in CD4 cells.[149,184] The exact nature of the immune response is not defined but cell mediated immunity is thought to play a key role. The means by which HIV brings about the progressive destruction of the immune system is unknown but the number of possible mechanisms include direct killing of cells by the virus,[218] syncytia formation,[173] autoimmune effects, infection and destruction of stem cells and destruction of normal immune regulatory pathways.[219,220] An underlying aspect of this process is virus load and a progressive disruption of the architecture of the immune organs.[61,184] While there is often an increase in virus load in the endstages of HIV infection and there is increasing evidence for virus replication in every stage of the disease[61,163,184] the level of circulating virus in the peripheral blood is relatively stable over considerable periods following the initial burst of viremia at the beginning of infection.[122] The level of persistent viremia has recently emerged as a major predictor of subsequent time to AIDS.[138,231] Those with a high baseline level of virus have a more rapid progression while those with a lower virus load have a longer AIDS-free survival and those who are stable, long-term survivors without evidence of progression have the lowest virus load.[141] The determinants of virus load are also unknown but probably involve host genetic factors as well as characteristics of the virus phenotype which may reflect growth characteristics of the virus.[10] The means by which the host immune system regulates virus load is not fully understood but here too immunogenetic factors may be important.[9] Cell mediated immunity may be a major determinant of infection. Other factors involved in disease progression are reflected in increasing virus load in lymph nodes and the disruption of lymph node cytoarchitecture particularly of the follicular dendritic cells.[66,185]

The timing of infection and subsequent disease progression varies between individuals.[127] In general, when a person is exposed to infectious virus, HIV p24 antigen is detectable within 4 to 6 weeks followed shortly thereafter by the appearance of antibody.[160] There are occasional instances where HIV virus has been detected in the absence of antibodies by virus culture or through the application of the polymerase chain reaction (PCR) amplification technique[112,170] although these instances are rare.[142] In some cases, exposed individuals have detectable cell mediated immunity in the absence of detectable virus or antibody, and these cases may represent exposure without infection or effective clearing of an abortive infection.[183] An acute viral syndrome has been reported among persons undergoing seroconversion. The incidence of this clinical syndrome characterized as a "flu-like" syndrome with fever, rash, myalgias, mouth sores and occasionally reversible encephalitis is not known but may be as high as 60%.[44] However, the symptoms are not specific enough to distinguish the acute illness for a variety of viral syndromes and thus these symptoms may or may not bring a patient to medical attention.[44] Following infection there is a long latent period sometimes associated with lymphadenopathy but often asymptomatic characterized by subclinical declines in CD-4 cells and perturbations in a number of other markers of immune function.[47,52,184,231] Epidemiologic studies have provided median estimates of the incubation time from HIV infection to clinical AIDS which vary between 8 to 10 years or more depending upon the age of the population studied, the precision of the window of seroconversion, and the nature of the exposure group.[19,24] Figure 10A/B portrays a more rapid progression to clinical AIDS by gay men than adult hemophiliacs. This may be explained in part by Kaposi sarcoma (KS) which almost exclusively occurs in gay men and often at a level of immune dysfunction less severe than seen with AIDS-associated opportunistic infections. There is a residual difference which may reflect differences in time to AIDS between risk groups. In addition there is some speculation that time to AIDS is more rapid in HIV–1 infected patients in developing countries where

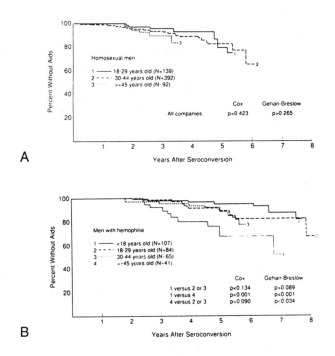

Figure 10A/B   AIDS incubation grouped by age at the time of seroconversion. A) AIDS incubation among gay men. (1) 18–29 years of age (solid line); 30–44 years of age (dashed line); (3) >44 years of age (dotted line). B) AIDS incubation among adult hemophiliacs. (1) < 18 years of age (solid line); (2) 18–29 years of age (dashed line); (3) 3–44 years of age (dotted line); (4) > 44 (thin solid line). Reproduced with permission from reference 20.

poor nutrition and other factors may influence immune response to virus infection.[162,217] Age at infection is the single most important determinant of time to AIDS in hemophiliacs (Figure 10B); persons infected in pre-adolescence and young adulthood progress much less rapidly from infection to AIDS than those who are infected after the age of 45.[19]

Children infected in the neonatal period have a more complex pattern of progression to AIDS. In a significant proportion of perinatally infected children the time to clinical AIDS defining illness is a matter of weeks to several months with a significant proportion developing disease by 6 months of age.[242,243] Another subset develop disease within the first 24 months of life, while a third group continue to survive for longer periods of time; the median incubation period is not yet defined.[113] The reasons for this variation in time to end stage immune dysfunction in infants is not known but variation in time of infection (e.g., prenatal versus perinatal), viral load, and viral strain have been conjectured.[165] Studies comparing the rate of progression of HIV infected children and adults have revealed that the time from exposure to depressed CD-4 lymphocyte count (e.g., <200 per mm^3) occurs more rapidly in adults over the age of 30 compared to the rate in children, adolescents, and young adults.[65,187] Furthermore, once this level of depression occurs the time to clinical immune dysfunction manifested as an AIDS defining illness is considerably more rapid in older adults than in younger persons.[89] Why age is such an important modifier of the natural history of HIV is unclear;[204] it may be a function of differences in the "reverse" of the immune system or a consequence of a yet-to-be-understood aspect of the host response where the virus is more effectively held in check during the early asymptomatic phase of infection. These findings have significant implications, not only to understanding the pathogenesis of HIV but also to evaluating therapy and other interventions where age may impact on outcome. Race does not appear to significantly influence time to AIDS[48] although some studies do suggest a more rapid progression from infection to AIDS in Africa.[60]

A role for coincident infections with other viruses as an accelerator of HIV progression has been a source of much debate based largely on *in vitro* studies of cell killing of HIV infected cells by a number of DNA viruses and the HTLV–I oncornavirus. Cytomegalovirus has been implicated as a cofactor in some studies[60] but not confirmed in others. Human herpes virus 6 (HIV 6) has also been considered without evidence of a clear association. The HTLV–I virus is associated with more rapid progression to AIDS in some cross-sectional studies; this may be a presentation of the immunostimulatory effects of HTLV–I on T-lymphocytes.[15] No such effect has been reported for HTLV–II. Mycoplasma have been implicated based on experimental studies, but no epidemiologic data nor positive benefit of intervention with suitable antibodies has been documented.[146,249]

High serum neopterin and B–2 microglobulin levels are examples of immune activation markers which predict progression to AIDS independent of CD–4 level.[43,131,189] Levels of antibody to the p24 antigen of HIV and free p24 antigen measure both the effectiveness of immune response to the virus and serves as a marker of free virus.[64,89] Quantitative measures of virus through culture and more recently PCR are independent measures of virus load which correlate with advanced stage of AIDS.[107] Recent prospective data from studies of exposure to AIDS have suggested that the level of immunity to virus (e.g., low p24 antibody response to HIV) and elevated virus load early in the course of infection, identify individuals at highest risk for subsequent progression to AIDS.[159] It is possible that the interaction between host immunity and perhaps host immunogenetic determinants of immune response as suggested by some studies, coupled with variations in virus strain result in heightened susceptibility for disease progression.[220] Further opportunity exists to investigate these factors in an effort to find a more precise means for identifying those most likely to benefit from early intervention with antiretroviral or immune modulating therapy, and to gain new insights of how some exposed persons hold the virus in check. Such investigations may provide an explanation which significantly advances our knowledge of HIV pathogenesis and infection therapy.

Summary and conclusions

From a public health perspective the HTLV and HIV viruses present markedly different patterns of occurrence and disease. HTLV–I and HTLV–II are endemic viruses; they occur worldwide and affect an estimated million or more persons. They cause disabling and sometimes fatal diseases, but this is rare. They provide a powerful model system for understanding the role of human retroviruses in cancer and other autoimmune type conditions with latency periods ranging from years to decades. These understudied viruses are an important tool for understanding the pathogenesis of a variety of chronic illnesses and it is likely that additional viruses of this class will be discovered in association with various diseases of unknown etiology.

The HIV/AIDS virus is spread by high risk behaviors and is at the center of a worldwide pandemic of unprecedented proportions; the fatality and morbidity rates are high, placing a strain on medical resources. The health care costs in the United States alone is currently approaching the trillion dollar mark (903.3 billion dollars; 14.4% of Gross Domestic Product (GDP)).[1] In the rest of the world, where 13 million are already infected and twice that number is projected by the end of the decade, the outlook is even more daunting.[1] The prognosticators anticipate widespread social and economic distress; they predict negative population curves and economic ruin in some countries.

A major thrust of current research efforts includes the development of an effective HIV–1 vaccine and the formulation of effective behavior interventions. If successful, these initiatives will provide future immunity and self-determined prevention; in either case, they should slacken the pace of virus propagation. Equally important are effective and affordable treatments for the millions of already infected persons at high risk for developing AIDS. Unfortunately the HIV virus has become a formidable foe; its high mutation rate allows circumvention of immunologic safeguards and resistance to drug therapies. The current debate considers how to allocate future research dollars and to decide what proportion should be dedicated to fundamental basic research, to applied treatment research, and to epidemiologic/molecular epidemiologic research.

References

1. AIDS in the world. In: Mann J., Tarantola, D. J. M., Netter T. W., eds. Cambridge, Massachusetts and London, England: Howard University Press. 1992:1–1037.
2. Aboulker, J. P., Swart, A. M. (1993). Preliminary analysis of the Concorde trial. *Lancet 341*:889–890.
3. Allen S., Serufilira, A., Gruber, V., et al. (1993). Pregnancy and contraception use among urban Rwandan women after HIV testing and counseling. *Am. J. Publ. Hlth. 83*:705–710.
4. Allen, S., Tice, J., Van de Perre P., et al. (1992). Effect of serotesting with counselling on condom use and seroconversion among HIV discordant couples in Africa. *Br. Med. J. 304*:1605–1609.
5. Anderson, R. M., May, R. M., Boily, M. C., Garnett, G. P., Rowley, J. T. (1991). The spread of HIV-1 in Africa: Sexual contact patterns and the predicted demographic impact of AIDS. *Nature 352*:581–589.

6. Anderson, R. M., May, R. M. McLean, A. R. (1988). Possible demographic consequences of AIDS in developing countries. *Nature 332*:228–234.
7. Ando Y., Nakano, S., Saito, K., et al. (1987). Transmission of adult T-cell leukemia retrovirus (HTLV-I) from mother to child: comparison of bottle-with breast-fed babies. *Japan J. Cancer Res. 78*:322–324.
8. Andrada-Serpa, M. J., Tosswill, J., Schor, D., Linhares, D., Dobbin, J., Pereira M. S. (1989). Seroepidemiologic survey for antibodies to human retroviruses in human and non-human primates in Brazil. *Int. J. Cancer 44*:389–393.
9. Ascher, M. S., Sheppard H. W. (1991). A unified hypothesis for three cardinal features of HIV immunology. *J. Acquir. Immune Defic. Syndr. 4*:97–98.
10. Ascher, M. S., Sheppard, H. W., Arnon, J. M., Lang, W. (1991). Viral burden in HIV disease. *J. Acquir. Immune Defic. Syndr. 4*:824–825.
11. Asou, N., Kumagai, T., Uekihara, S., et al. (1986). HTLV-I seroprevalence in patients with malignancy. *Cancer, 58*:903–907.
12. Baltimore, D. (1970). RNA-dependent DNA polymerase in virions of RNA tumor viruses. *Nature 226*:1209–1211.
13. Barre-Sinoussi, F., Chermann, J.-C., Rey F., et al. (1983). Isolation of a T-lymphotropic retrovirus from a patient at risk for acquired immune deficiency syndrome (AIDS). *Science 220*:868–871.
14. Bartholomew, C., Cleghorn, F. R., Blattner, W. A. (1988). HTLV-I as a cofactor in AIDS. In Watson R., ed. Cofactors in human immunodeficiency virus, infection and progression to AIDS. Boca Raton, FL: CRC Press, 147–150.
15. Bartholomew, C., Saxinger, C. W., Clark, J. W., et al. (1987). Transmission of HTLV-I and HIV among homosexual men in Trinidad. *J. Am. Med. Assoc. 257*: 2604–2608.
16. Bastian, I., Gardner, J., Webb, D., Gardner, I. (1993). Isolation of a human T-lymphotropic virus type I strain from Australian aboriginals. *J. Virol. 6*:843–851.
17. Benveniste, R. E. (1985). The contributions of retroviruses to the study of mammalian evolution. In MacIntyre, R. J., ed. Molecular evolutionary genetics. Plenum Publishing Corporation, 359–417.
18. Berneman, A., Gartenhaus, R. B., Reitz, M. S., Jr. (1992). Expression of alternatively spliced human T-lymphotropic virus type I px mRNA in infected cell lines and in primary uncultured cells from patients with adult T-cell leukemia/lymphoma and healthy carriers. *Proc. Natl. Acad. Sci. USA 89*:3005–3009.
19. Biggar, R. J. (1990). International Registry of Seroconverters. AIDS incubation in 1891 HIV seroconverters from different exposure groups. *AIDS 4*:1059–1066.
20. Blanche, S., Rouzioux, C., Moscato, M. L., et al. (1989). A prospective study of infants born to women seropositive for human immunodeficiency virus type 1. *N. Engl. J. Med. 320*: 1643–1648.
21. Blattner, W. A. (1989). Retroviruses. In Evans A. S. ed. Viral infections of human epidemiology and control. 3rd ed. New York: Plenum Medical Press. 545–592.
22. Blattner, W. A., Gibbs, W. N., Saxinger, C. W., et al. (1983). Human T-cell leukemia/lymphoma virus-associated lymphoreticular neoplasia in Jamaica. *Lancet* 2:61–64.

23. Blattner, W. A., Kalyanaraman, V. S., Robert-Guroff, M. et al. (1982). The human type-C retrovirus, HTLV, in blacks from the Caribbean region, and relationship to adult T-cell leukemia/lymphoma. *Int. J. Cancer 30*:257–264.

24. Blaxhult, A., Granath, F., Kidman, K., Giesecke, J. (1990). The influence of age on the latency period to AIDS in people infected by HIV through blood transfusion. *AIDS 4*:125–129.

25. Bowler, S., Sheon, A. R., D'Angelo, L. J., Vermund, S. H. (1992). HIV and AIDS among adolescents in the United States: increasing risk in the 1990s. *J. Adolesc 15*:345–371.

26. Brookmeyer, R. (1991). Reconstruction and future trends of the AIDS epidemic in the United States. *Science 253*:37–42.

27. Brundage, J. F., Burke, D. S., Gardner, L. I., et al. (1990). Tracking the spread of the HIV infection epidemic among young adults in the United States: results of the first four years of screening among civilian applicants for U.S. military service. *J. Acquir. Immune Defic. Syndr. 3*:1168–1180.

28. Cartier, L., Araya, F., Castillo, J. L. (1993). Southernmost carriers of HTLV-I/II in the world. *Jap. J. Cancer Res. 84*:1–3.

29. Catovsky, D., Greaves, M. F. (1982). Adult T-cell lymphoma-leukaemia in blacks form the West Indies. *Lancet 1*:639–643.

30. Centers for Disease Control (1981). Pneumocystis pneumonia—Los Angeles. *MMWR Morb. Mortal. Wkly. Rep. 30*:250–252.

31. Centers for Disease Control (1987). Update: human immunodeficiency virus infections in health-care workers exposed to blood of infected patients. *MMWR Morb. Mortal. Wkly. Rep. 36*:285–289.

32. Centers for Disease Control (1990). Human T-lymphotropic virus type I screening in volunteer blood donors: United States, 1989. *MMWR Morb. Mortal. Wkly. Rep. 39*:915–925.

33. Centers for Disease Control (1991). Patterns of sexual behavior change among homosexual/bisexual men—selected U.S. sites, 1987–1990. *MMWR Morb. Mortal. Wkly. Rep. 40*:792–794.

34. Centers for Disease Control (1991). Mortality attributable to HIV infection/AIDS—United States, 1981–1990. *MMWR Morb. Mortal. Wkly. Rep. 40*:41–44.

35. Centers for Disease Control (1991). Opportunistic non-Hodgkin's lymphomas among severely immunocompromised HIV-infected patients-surviving for prolonged periods on antiretroviral therapy-United States. *MMWR Morb. Mortal. Wkly. Rep. 40*:591–601.

36. Centers for Disease Control (1991). The HIV/AIDS epidemic: the first 10 years. *MMWR Morb. Mortal. Wkly. Rep. 40*:357.

37. Centers for Disease Control (1992). Surveillance for occupationally acquired HIV infection—United States, 1981–1992. *MMWR Morb. Mortal. Wkly. Rep. 41*:823–825.

38. Centers for Disease Control (1993). Up-date: Barrier Protection Against HIV Infection and other Sexually Transmitted Diseases. *MMWR Morb. Mortal. Wkly. Rep. 42*:589–597.

39. Centers for Disease Control (1993). Update: Acquired Immunodeficiency Syndrome—United States, 1992. *MMWR Morb. Mortal. Wkly. Rep. 42*:547–557.

40. Cheng-Mayer, C., Seto, D., Tateno, M., Levy, J. A. (1988). Biologic features of HIV-1 that correlate with virulence in the host. *Science 240*:80–82.

41. Clark, J., Saxinger, C. W., Gibbs, W. N., et al. (1985). Seroepidemiologic studies of human T-cell leukemia/lymphoma virus type I in Jamaica. *Int. J. Cancer 36*:37–41.

42. Clark, J. W., Robert-Guroff, M., Ikehara, O., Henzan, E., Blattner, W. A. (1985). Human T-cell leukemia-lymphoma virus type 1 and adult T-cell leukemia-lymphoma in Okinawa. *Int. J. Cancer 45*:2849–2852.

43. Colton, T., Freedman, L. S., Johnson, A. L., Machin, D. (1993). Markers paths. In Gore S. M. Farewell, V. T., eds. Statistics in medicine. John Wiley & Sons, 2099–2126.

44. Cooper, D. A., Gold, J., MacLean, P., et al. (1985). Acute AIDS retrovirus infection. Definition of a clinical illness associated with seroconversion. *Lancet 1*:537–540.

45. Corbitt, G., Bailey, A. S., Williams, G. (1990). HIV infection in Manchester, 1959. *Lancet 336*:51.

46. Cossen C., Hagens, S., Fukuchi, R., Forghani, B., Gallo, D., Ascher, M. (1992). Comparison of six commercial human T-cell lymphotropic virus type I (HTLV-I) enzyme immunoassay kits for detection of antibody to HTLV-I and -II. *J. Clin. Microbiol. 30*:724–725.

47. Crowe, S. M., Carlin, J. B., Stewart, K. I., Lucas, C. R., Hoy, J. F. (1991). Predictive value of CD4 lymphocyte numbers for the development of opportunistic infections and malignancies in HIV-infected persons. *J. Acquir. Immune Defic. Syndr. 4*:770–776.

48. Curtis, J. R., Patrick, D. L. (1993). Race and Survival time with AIDS: a synthesis of the literature. *Am. J. Public Health 83*:1425–1428.

49. Daar, E. S., Moudgil, T., Meyer, R. D., Ho, D. D. (1991). Transient high levels of viremia in patients with primary human immunodeficiency virus type 1 infection. *N. Engl. J. Med. 324*:961–964.

50. Dada, A. J., Oyewole, F., Onofowokan, R., et al. (1993). Demographic characteristics of retroviral infections (HIV-1, HIV-2 and HTLV-I) among female professional sex workers in Lagos, Nigeria. *J. Acquir. Immune Defic. Syndr. 6*:1358–1363.

51. Dalgleish, A. G., Beverley, P. C., Clapham, P. R., Crawford, D. H., Greaves, M. F., Weiss, R. A. (1984). The CD4 (T4) antigen is an essential component of the receptor for the AIDS retrovirus. *Nature 312*:763–767.

52. Dawson, J. D., Lagakos, S. W. (1991). Analyzing laboratory marker changes in AIDS clinical trials. *J. Acquir. Immune Defic. Syndr. 4*:667–676.

53. De Cock, K. M., Barrere, B., Diaby, L., et al. (1990). AIDS—the leading cause of adult death in the West African City of Abidjan, Ivory Coast. *Science 249*:793–796.

54. De-Thé G., Giordano, C., Gessain, A., et al. (1989). Human retroviruses HTLV-I, HIV-1, and HIV-2 and neurological diseases in some equatorial areas of Africa. *J. Acquir. Immune Defic. Syndr.* 2:550–556.
55. Des Jarlais, D. C., Friedman, S. R. (1988). HIV infection among persons who inject illicit drugs: problems and perspectives. *J. Acquir. Immune Defic. Syndr.* 1:267–273.
56. Des Jarlais, D. C., Friedman, S. R., Novick, D. M., et al. (1989). HIV-I infection among intravenous drug users in Manhattan, New York City, from 1977 through 1987. *J. Am. Med. Assoc.* 261:1008–1012.
57. Di Rienzo, A. M., Petronini, P. G., Guetard, D., et al. (1992). Modulation of cell growth and host protein synthesis during HIV infection *in vitro*. *J. Acquir. Immune Defic. Syndr.* 5:921–929.
58. Donegan, E. A., Lenes, B. A., Tomasulo, P. A., Mosely, J. W. (1990). Transmission of HIV-1 by component type and duration of shelf storage before transfusion. *Transfusion 30*:851–852.
59. Donegan, E. A., Stuart, M., Niland, J. C., et al. (1990). Infection with human immunodeficiency virus type 1 (HIV-1) among recipients of antibody-positive blood donations. *Ann. Intern. Med.* 113:733–739.
60. Drew, W. L. (1986). Is cytomegalovirus a cofactor in the pathogenesis of AIDS and Kaposi's Sarcoma. *Mt. Sinai J. Med.* 53:622–626.
61. Embretson, J., Zupancic, M., Ribas, J. L., et al. (1993). Massive covert infection of helper T lymphocytes and macrophages by HIV during the incubation period of AIDS. *Nature 362*:359–362.
62. Essex, M., Kanki, P. J. (1988). The origins of the AIDS virus. The AIDS virus is not unique. It has relatives in man as well as other primates. Studies of related viruses indicate that some have evolved disease-free coexistence with their animal hosts. *Sci. Am.* 64–71.
63. Eyster, M. E., Alter, H. J., Aledort, L. M., Quan, S., Hatzakis, A., Goedert, J. J. (1991). Heterosexual co-transmission of hepatitis C virus (HCV) and human immunodeficiency virus (HIV). *Ann. Intern. Med.* 115:764–768.
64. Eyster, M. E., Ballard, J. O., Gail, M. H., Drumond, J. E., Goedert, J. J. (1989). Predictive markers for the acquired immunodeficiency syndrome (AIDS) in hemophiliacs: persistence of p24 antigen and low T4 cell count. *Ann. Intern. Med.* 110:963–969.
65. Eyster, M. E., Rabkin, C. S., Hilgartner, M. W. et al. (1993). Human immunodeficiency virus-related conditions in children and adults with hemophilia: rates, relationship to CD4 counts, and predictive value. *Blood 81*:828–834.
66. Fauci, A., Schnittman, S. M., Poli, G., Koenig, S., Pantaleo, G. (1991). Immunopathogenetic mechanisms in human immunodeficiency virus (HIV) infection. *Ann. Intern. Med.* 114:678–693.
67. Figueroa, J. P., Brathwaite, A., Morris, J., et al. (1994). Rising HIV-1 prevalence among sexually transmitted disease clinic attenders in Jamaica: traumatic sex and genital ulcers as risk factors. *J. Acquir. Immune Defic. Syndr.* 7:310–316.

68. Fine, H. A., Mayer, R. J. (1993). Primary central nervous system lymphoma. *Ann. Intern. Med. 119*:1093–1104.
69. Flugel, R. M. (1991). Spumaviruses: a group of complex retroviruses. *J. Acquir. Immune Defic. Syndr. 4*:739–750.
70. Gabriel, V., Packham, D. R. (1993). Heterosexual transmission: a growing risk factor for HIV spread. *Aust. N. Z. J. Obstet. Gynaecol. 33*:174–176.
71. Gail, M. H., Pluda, J. M., Rabkin, C. S., et al. (1991). Projections of the incidence of non-Hodgkin's lymphoma related to acquired immunodeficiency syndrome. *J. Natl. Cancer Inst. 83*:695–701.
72. Gail, M. H., Rosenberg, P. S., Goedert, J. J. (1990). Therapy may explain recent deficits in AIDS incidence. *J. Acquir. Immune Defic. Syndr. 3*:296–306.
73. Gallo, R., Wong-Staal, F., Montagnier, L., Haseltine, W. A., Yoshida, M. ((1988). HIV/HTLV gene nomenclature. *Nature 333*:504.
74. Gallo, R. C. (1991). Mechanism of disease induction by HIV. *J. Acquir Immune Defic. Syndr. 3*:380–389.
75. Gallo, R. C. (1991). Human retroviruses: a decade of discovery and link with human disease. *J. Infect Dis. 164*:235–243.
76. Gallo, R. C., Wong-Staal, F., Sarin, P. S. (1989). Cellular ONC genes, T-cell leukaemia-lymphoma virus, and leukaemias and lymphomas of man. *Mech. Viral Leukaemogenesis,* 11–37.
77. Gao, F., Yue, L., White, A. T., et al. (1992). Human infection by genetically diverse SIV related HIV-2 in West Africa. *Nature 358*:495–499.
78. Garruto, R. M., Slover, M., Yanagihara, R., et al. (1990). High prevalence of human T-lymphotropic virus type I infection in isolated populations of the Western Pacific region confirmed by Western immunoblot. *Am. J. Hum. Biol. 2*:439–447.
79. Gayle, H., Jnaore, E., Adjorlolo, G., Ekpini, E., Porter, A., DeCock, K. M. (1989). HIV infection in children, Abidjan, Cote d'Ivoire. *Epidemiology, F*-1:33.
80. Gessain, A., Barin, F., Vernant, J. C., et al. (1985). Antibodies to human T-lymphotropic virus type-I in patients with tropical spastic paraparesis. *Lancet* 2:407–410.
81. Gessain, A., Boeri, E., Yanagihara, R., Gallo, R. C., Franchini, G. (1993). Complete nucleotide sequence of a highly divergent human T-cell leukemia (lymphotropic) virus type I (HTLV-I) variant from Melanesia: genetic and phylogenetic relationship to HTLV-I strains from other geographical regions. *J. Virol. 67*: 1015–1023.
82. Gessain, A., Caudie, C., Gout, O., et al. (1988). Intrathecal synthesis of antibodies to human T lymphotropic virus type I and the presence of IgG oligoclonal bands in the cerebrospinal fluid of patients with endemic tropical spastic paraparesis. *J. Infect. Dis. 157*:1226–1234.
83. Gessain, A., Francis, H., Sonan, T., et al. (1986). HTLV-I and tropical spastic paraparesis in Africa. *Lancet 1*:698.
84. Gessain, A., Fretz, C., Koulibaly, M., et al. (1993). Evidence of HTLV-II infection in Guinea, West Africa. *J. Acquir. Immune Defic. Syndr. 6*:324–325.

85. Gessain, A., Tuppin, P., Kazanji, M., et al. (1994). A distinct molecular variant of HTLV-IIB in Gabon, Central Africa. *AIDS Res. Hum. Retroviruses 10*:753–755.

86. Gilks, C. F. (1993). The clinical challenge of the HIV epidemic in the developing world. *Lancet 342*:1037–1039.

87. Goedert, J. J., Blattner, W. A. (1988). The epidemiology and natural history of human immunodeficiency virus. In: Devita, V. T., Hellman, S., Rosenberg, S. A., eds. AIDS: etiology, diagnosis, treatment and prevention. 2nd ed. Philadelphia: V. P. Lippincott Co., 33–60.

88. Goedert, J. J., Eyster, M. E., Biggar, R. J., Blattner, W. A. (1987). Heterosexual transmission of human immunodeficiency virus: association with severe depletion of T-helper lymphocytes in men with hemophilia. *AIDS Res. Hum. Retroviruses, 3*:355–361.

89. Goedert, J. J., Kessler, C. M., Aledort, L. M., et al. (1989). A prospective study of human immunodeficiency virus type 1 infection and the development of AIDS in subjects with hemophilia. *N. Engl. J. Med. 321*:1141–1148.

90. Goedert, J. J., Mendez, H., Drummond, J. E., et al. (1989). Mother-to-infant transmission of human immunodeficiency virus type 1: association with prematurity or low anti-gp120. *Lancet 2*:1351–1355.

91. Goubau, P., Desmyter, J., Ghesquiere, J., Kasereka, B. (1992). HTLV-II among pygmies. *Nature 359*:201.

92. Gracia, F., Reeves, W. C., Levine, P. H., et al. (1990). Human T-cell lymphotropic virus type I and neurologic disease in Panama, 1985 and 1986. *Arch. Neurol. 47*:634–639.

93. Greaves, M. F., Colman, S. M., Beard, M. E. J., et al. (1993). Geographical distribution of acute lymphoblastic leukaemia subtypes: second report of the collaborative group study. *Leukemia, 7*:27–34.

94. Green, T. A., Karon, J. M., Nwanyanwu, O. C. (1992). Changes in AIDS incidence trends in the United States. *J. Acquir. Immune Defic. Syndr. 5*:547–555.

95. Hague, R. A., Mok, J. Y. Q., Johnstone, F. D., et al. (1993). Maternal factors in HIV transmission. *Int. J. STD. AIDS 4*:142–146.

96. Hall, W. W., Liu, C. R., Scheenwind, O., et al. (1991). Deleted HTLV-I provirus in blood and cutaneous lesions of patients with mycosis fungoides. *Science 253*:317–320.

97. Hall, W. W., Takahashi, H., Liu, C., et al. (1992). Multiple isolates and characteristics of human T-cell leukemia virus type II. *J. Virol. 66*:2456–2463.

98. Hall, W. W., Zhu, S. W., Horal, P., Furuta, Y., Zagaany, G., Vahine, A. (1994). HTLV-II infection in Mongolia. *AIDS Res. Hum. Retroviruses, 10*:443. (abstract)

99. Hanchard, B., LaGrenade, L., Carberry, C., et al. (1991). Childhood infective dermatitis evolving into adult T-cell leukaemia after 17 years. [Letter]. *Lancet 338*:1593–1594.

100. Hartley, T. M., Malone, G. E., Khabbaz, R. F., Lal, R. B., Kaplan, J. E. (1991). Evaluation of a recombinant human T-cell lymphotropic virus type I (HTLV-I) p21E antibody detection enzyme immunoassay as a supplementary test in HTLV-I/II antibody testing algorithms. *J. Clin. Microbiol. 29*:1125–1127.

101. Heneine, W., Kaplan, J. E., Gracia, F., et al. (1991). HTLV-II endemicity among Guaymi Indians in Panama. [Letter]. *N. Engl. J. Med. 324*: 565.
102. Heneine, W., Khabbaz, R. F., Lal, R. B., Kaplan, J. E. (1992). Sensitive and specific polymerase chain reaction assays for diagnosis of human T-cell lymphotropic virus type I (HTLV-I) and HTLV-II infections in HTLV-I/II-seropositive individuals. *J. Clin. Microbiol. 30*:1605–1607.
103. Hino, S. (1990). Maternal-infant transmission of HTLV-I implication for disease. In: Blattner, W. A., ed. *Human Retrovirology (HTLV-I)*. New York: Raven Press, 363–375.
104. Hinuma, Y., Komoda, H., Chosa, T., et al. (1982). Antibodies to adult T-cell leukemia virus-associated antigen (ATLA) in sera from patients with ATL and controls in Japan: A nation-wide sero-epidemiologic study. *Int. J. Cancer, 29*:631–635.
105. Hjelle, B., Appenzeller, O., Mills, R., et al. (1992). Chronic neurodegenerative disease associated with HTLV-II infection. *Lancet, 339*:645–646.
106. Hjelle, B., Scalf, R., Swenson, S. (1990). High frequency of human T-cell leukemia-lymphoma virus type II infection in New Mexico blood donors: determination by sequence-specific oligonucleotide hybridization. *Blood, 76*:450–454.
107. Ho, D. D., Moudgil, T., Alam, M. (1989). Quantitation of human immunodeficiency virus type I in the blood of infected persons. *N. Engl. J. Med. 321*:1621–1625.
108. Hoover, D. R., Graham, N. M. H., Chen B., et al. (1992). Effect of CD4+ cell count measurement variability on staging HIV-1 infection. *J. Acquir. Immune Defic. Syndr. 5*:794–802.
109. Hser, Y. I. (1993). Population estimates of intravenous drug users and HIV infection in Los Angeles County. *Int. J. Addict 28*: 695–709.
110. Ichimaru, M., Ikeda, S., Kinoshita, K., Hino, S., Tsuji, Y. (1991). Mother-to-child transmission of HTLV-I. *Cancer Detect. Prev. 15*:177–181.
111. Igichi, S., Ramundo, M. B., Takahashi, H., Hall, W. W. (1992). *In vivo* cellular trophisms of human T-cell leukemia virus type II (HTLV II). *J. Exp. Med. 176*:293–296.
112. Imagawa, D. T., Lee M. H., Wolinsky, S. M., et al. (1989). Human immunodeficiency virus type 1 infection in homosexual men who remain seronegative for prolonged periods. *N. Engl. J. Med. 320*:1458–1462.
113. Italian Registry HIV Infection in Children (1994). Features of children perinatally infected with HIV-1 surviving longer than 5 years. *Lancet 343*:191–195.
114. Jacobson, S., Lehky, T., Nishimura, M., Robinson, S., McFarlin, D., Dhib-Jalbut, S. (1993). Isolation of HTLV-II from a patient with chronic, progressive neurological disease clinically indistinguishable from HTLV-I-associated myelopathy/tropical spastic paraparesis. *Am. Neur. Assoc. 14*:392–396.
115. Jacobson, S., Shida, H., McFarlin, D. E., Fauci, A. S., Koenig, S. (1990). Circulating CD8+ cytotoxic T lymphocytes specific for HTLV-I pX in patients with HTLV-I associated neurological disease. *Nature 348*:245–248.
116. Johnson, A. M., Petherick, A., Davidson, S. J., et al. (1989). Transmission of HIV to heterosexual partners of infected men and women. *AIDS 3*:367–372.

117. Johnson, A. M., Wadsworth, J., Wellings, K.., Bradshaw, S., Field, J. (1992). Sexual lifestyles and HIV risk. *Nature* 360:410–412.
118. Kajiyama, W., Kashiwagi, S., Ikematsu, H., Hayashi, J., Nomura, H., Okochi, K. (1986). Intrafamilial transmission of adult T cell leukemia virus. *J. Infect. Dis.* 154:851–857.
119. Kajiyama, W., Kashiwagi, S., Nomura, H., Ikematsu, H., Hayashi, J., Ikematsu, W. (1986). Seroepidemiologic study of antibody to adult T-cell leukemia virus in Okinawa. *Japan Am. J. Epidemiol.* 123:41–47.
120. Kalyanaraman, V. S., Sarngadharan, M. G., Robert-Guroff, M., et al. (1982). A new subtype of human T-cell leukemia virus (HTLV-II) associated with a T-cell variant of hairy cell leukemia. *Science,* 218:571–573.
121. Kanki, P., Essex, M. (1988). Simian T-lymphotropic viruses and related human viruses. *Vet. Microbiol.* 17:309–314.
122. Katzenstein, D. A., Holodniy, M., Israelski, D. M., et al. (1992). Plasma viremia in human immunodeficiency virus infection: relationship to stage of disease and antiviral treatment. *J. Acquir. Immune Defic. Syndr.* 5:107–112.
123. Khabbaz, R. F., Rowe, T., Murphey-Corb, M., et al. (1992). Simian immunodeficiency virus needlestick accident in a laboratory worker. *Lancet* 340:271–273.
124. Killewo, J. Z. J., Sandstrom, A., Raden, U. B., Mhalu, F. S., Biberfeld, G., Wall, S. (1993). Incidence of HIV-1 infection among adults in the Kagera region of Tanzania. *Int. J. Epidemiol.* 22:528–536.
125. Kinoshita, K., Amagasaki, T., Hino, S., et al. (1987). Milk-borne transmission of HTLV-I from carrier mothers to their children. *Japan J. Cancer Res.* 78:674–680.
126. Kong, L. I., Lee, S., Kappes, J. C., et al. (1988). West African HIV-2-related human retrovirus with attenuated cytopathicity. *Science,* 240:1525–1529.
127. Krämer, A., Biggar, R. J., Hampl, H., et al. (1992). Immunologic markers of progression to acquired immunodeficiency syndrome are time-dependent and illness-specific. *Am. J. Epidemiol.* 136:71–80.
128. Krämer, A., Jacobson, S., Reuben, J. S., et al. (1990). Spontaneous lymphocyte proliferation is elevated in asymptomatic HTLV-I-positive Jamaicans. In Blattner, W. A., ed. *Human Retrovirology: HTLV.* New York: Raven Press. 79–85.
129. Kreiss, J. K., Koech, D., Plummer, F. A., et al. (1986). AIDS virus infection in Nairobi prostitutes. Spread of the epidemic to East Africa. *N. Engl. J. Med.* 314:414–418.
130. Kroner, B. L., Rosenberg, P. S., Aledort, L. M., Alvord, W. G., Goedert, J. J. (1994). HIV-1 infection incidence among persons with hemophilia in the United States and Western Europe, 1978–1990. *J. Acquir. Immune Defic. Syndr.* 7:279–286.
131. Krown, S. E., Niedzwiecki, D., Bhalla, R. B., Flomenberg, N., Bundow, D., Chapman, D. (1991). Relationship and prognostic value of endogenous interferon-α. β-microglobulin, and neopterin serum levels in patients with Kaposi's sarcoma and AIDS. *J. Acquir. Immune Defic. Syndr.* 4:871–880.

132. LaGrenade, L., Hanchard, B., Fletcher, V., Cranston, B., Blattner, W. A. (1990). Infective dermatitis of Jamaican children: a marker for HTLV-I infection. *Lancet* *336*:1345–1346.

133. LaGrenade, L., Morgan, O., Carberry, C., et al. (1995). Tropical spastic paraparesis occurring in HTLV-I associated infective dermatitis: a report of two cases. *West Indian Med. J. 44*:34–35.

134. Lairmore, M. D., Jacobson, S., Gracia, F., et al. (1990). Isolation of human T-cell lymphotropic virus type 2 from Guaymi Indians in Panama. *Proc. Natl. Acad. Sci. USA 87*:8840–8844.

135. Lal, R. B., Brodine, S. K., Coligan, J. E., Roberts, C. R. (1991). Differential antibody responsiveness to p19 gag results in serological discrimination between human T lymphotropic virus type I and type II. *J. Med. Virol. 35*:232–236.

136. Le Pont, F., Valleron, A. J. (1993). Potential HIV epidemic associated with heterosexual transmission among youth in France. *AIDS 7*:1134–1135.

137. Lee, H. H., Swanson, P., Rosenblatt, J. D., et al. (1991). Relative prevalence and risk factors of HTLV-I and HTLV-II infection in US blood donors. *Lancet 337*:1435–1439.

138. Lee, T. H., Sheppard, H. W., Reis, M., Dondero, D., Osmond, D., Busch, M. P. (1994). Circulating HIV-1 infected cell burden from seroconversion to AIDS: importance of postseroconversion viral load on disease course. *J. Acquir. Immune Defic. Syndr. 7*:381–388.

139. Levine, A. M. (1991). Lymphoma related to human immunodeficiency virus: the epidemic shifts. *J. Natl. Cancer Inst. 83*:662–663.

140. Levine, P. H., Jacobson, S., Elliott, R., et al. (1993). HTLV-II infection in Florida Indians. *AIDS Res. Hum. Retroviruses 9*:123–127.

141. Lifson, A. R., Buchbinder, S. P., Sheppard, H. W., et al. (1991). Long-term human immunodeficiency virus infection in asymptomatic homosexual and bisexual men with normal CD4+ lymphocyte counts: immunologic and virologic characteristics. *J. Infect. Dis. 163*:959–965.

142. Lifson, A. R., Stanley, M., Pane, J., et al. (1990). Detection of human immunodeficiency virus DNA using the polymerase chain reaction in a well-characterized group of homosexual and bisexual men. *J. Infect. Dis. 161*:436–439.

143. Lillehoj, E. P., Alexander, S. S., Dubrule, C. J., et al. (1990). Development and evaluation of a human T-cell leukemia virus type I serologic confirmatory assay incorporating a recombinant envelope polypeptide. *J. Clin. Microbiol. 28*:2653–2658.

144. Lindan, C., Allen, S., Carael, M., et al. (1991). Knowledge, attitudes and perceived risk of AIDS among urban Rwandan women: relationship to HIV infection and behavior change. *AIDS 5*:993–1002.

145. Lipka, J. J., Santiago, P., Chan, L., et al. (1991). Modified western blot assay for confirmation and differentiation of human T-cell lymphotropic virus types I and II. *J. Infect. Dis. 164*:400–403.

146. Lo, S. C., Hayes, M. M., Wang, R. Y. H., Pierce, P. F., Kotani, H., Shih, J. W. K. (1991). Newly discovered mycoplasma isolated from patients infected with HIV. *Lancet 338*:1415–1418.

147. Loughran, T. P., Jr., Coyle, T., Sherman, M. P., et al. (1992). Detection of human T-cell leukemia/lymphoma virus, type II, in a patient with large granular lymphocyte leukemia. *Blood 80*:1116–1119.

148. Lu, W., Eme, D., Andrieu, J. M. (1993). HIV viraemia and seroconversion. *Lancet 341*:113.

149. Luzuriaga, K., McQuilken, P., Alimenti, A., Somasundaram, M., Hesselton, R. A., Sullivan, J. L. (1993). Early viremia and immune responses in vertical human immunodeficiency virus type 1 infection. *J. Infect Dis. 167*:1008–1013.

150. Madeleine, M. M. Wiktor, S. Z., Goedert, J. J., et al. (1993). HTLV-I and HTLV-II world-wide distribution: reanalysis of 4,832 immunoblot results. *Int. J. Cancer 54*:255–260.

151. Maloney, E. M., Biggar, R. J., Neel, J. V., et al. (1992). Endemic human T-cell lymphotropic virus type II infection among isolated Brazilian Amerindians. *J. Infect. Dis. 166*:100–107.

152. Mann, J. M. (1990). Global AIDS into the 1990s. *J. Acquir. Immune Defic. Syndr. 3*:438–442.

153. Manns, A., Murphy, E. L., Wilks, R., et al. (1989). Detection of early HTLV-I seroconversion (SC). *Seventh Int. Conf. AIDS 5*(B636):503. (abstract)

154. Manns, A., Wilks, R. J., Murphy, E. L., et al. (1992). A prospective study of transmission by transfusion of HTLV-I and risk factors associated with seroconversion. *Int. J. Cancer 51*:886–891.

155. Martin, M. P., Biggar, R. J., Hamlin-Green, G., Staal, S., Mann, D. (1993). Large granular lymphocytosis in a patient infected with HTLV-II. *AIDS Res. Hum. Retroviruses 9*:715–719.

156. Mastro, T. D., Satten, G. A., Nopkesorn, T., Sangkharomya, S., Longini, I. M., Jr. (1994). Probability of female-to-male transmission of HIV-1 in Thailand. *Lancet 343*:204–207.

157. Matsuzaki, H., Asou, N., Kawaguchi, Y. (1990). Human T-cell leukemia virus type I associated with small cell lung cancer. *Cancer 66*;1763–1768.

158. McCutchan, F. E., Ungar, B. L. P., Hegerich, P., et al. (1992). Genetic analysis of HIV-1 isolates from Zambia and an expanded phylogenetic tree for HIV-1. *J. Acquir. Immune Defic. Syndr. 5*:441–449.

159. McHugh, T. M., Stites, D. P., Busch, M. P., Krowka, J. F., Strickler, R. B., Hollander, H. (1988). Relation of circulating levels of human immunodeficiency virus (HIV) antigen, antibody to p24, and HIV-containing immune complexes in HIV-infected patients. *J. Infect Dis. 158*:1088–1091.

160. McRae, B., Lange, J. A. M., Ascher, M. S., et al. (1991). Immune response to HIV p24 core protein during the early phases of human immunodeficiency virus infection. *AIDS Res. Hum. Retroviruses 7*:637–643.

161. Meytes, D., Schochat, B., Lee, H., et al. (1990). Serological and molecular survey for HTLV-I infection in a high-risk middle eastern group. *Lancet 336*:1533–1535.

162. Mgone, C. S., Mhalu, F. S., Shao, J. F., et al. (1991). Prevalence of HIV-1 infection and symptomatology of AIDS in severely malnourished children in Dar Es Salaam, Tanzania. *J. Acquir. Immune Defic. Syndr. 4*:910–913.

163. Michael, N. L., Vahey, M., Burke, D. S., Redfield, R. R. (1992). Viral DNA and mRNA expression correlate with the stage of human immunodeficiency virus (HIV) type 1 infection in humans: Evidence for viral replication in all stages of HIV disease. *J. Virol. 66*:310–316.

164. Mochizuki, M., Watanabe, T., Yamaguchi, K., et al. (1992). Uveitis associated with human T-cell lymphotropic virus type I. *Am. J. Ophthalmol. 114*:123–129.

165. Mofenson, L. M., Blattner, W. A. (1992). Human retroviruses. In Feigin, R. D., Cherry, J. D., eds. Textbook of pediatric infectious diseases. 3rd ed. Philadelphia: W. B. Saunders Company, 1757–1788.

166. Morgan, O. S., Rodgers-Johnson, P., Mora, C., Char, G. (1989). HTLV-I and polymyositis in Jamaica. *Lancet 2*:1184–1187.

167. Murphy, E. L., Figueroa, J. P., Gibbs, W. N., et al. (1986). Sexual transmission of human T-lymphotropic virus type I (HTLV-I). *Ann. Intern. Med. 111*:555–560.

168. Nakano, S., Ando, Y., Saito, K., et al. (1986). Primary infection of Japanese infants with adult T-cell leukemia-associated retrovirus (ATLV): evidence for viral transmission from mothers to children. *J. Infect. 12*:205–212.

169. Nelson, K. E., Celentano, D. D., Suprasert, S., et al. (1993). Risk factors for HIV infection among young adult men in northern Thailand. *J. Am. Med. Assoc. 270*:955–960.

170. Nielsen, C., Teglbjaerg, L. S., Pedersen, C., Lundgren, J. D., Nielsen, C. M., Vestergaard, B. F. (1991). Prevalence of HIV infection in seronegative high-risk individuals examined by virus isolation and PCR. *J. Acquir. Immune Defic. Syndr. 4*:1107–1111.

171. Nishioka, K., Maruyama, I., Sato, K., Kitajima, I., Nakajima, Y., Osame, M. (1989). Chronic inflammatory arthropathy associated with HTLV-I. *Lancet 1*:441.

172. Nopkesorn, T., Mastro, T. D., Sangkharomya, S., et al. (1993). HIV-1 infection in young men in northern Thailand. *AIDS 7*:1233–1239.

173. Ohki, K., Kishi, M., Nishino, Y., et al. (1991). Noninfectious doughnut-shaped human immunodeficiency virus type 1 can induce syncytia mediated by fusion of the particles with CD4-positive cells. *J. Acquir. Immune Defic. Syndr. 4*:1233–1240.

174. Okamoto, T., Mori, S., Ohno, Y., et al. (1990). Stochastic analysis of the carcinogenesis of adult T-cell leukemia-lymphoma. In Blattner, W. A., ed. Human Retrovirology: HTLV. New York: Raven Press, 307–313.

175. Okamoto, T., Ohno, Y., Tsugane S., et al. (1989). Multi-step carcinogenesis model for adult T-cell leukemia. *Japan J. Cancer Res. 80*:191–195.

176. Okayama, A., Chen, Y. A., Tachibana, N., et al. (1991). High incidence of antibodies to HTLV-I tax in blood relatives of adult T cell leukemia patients. *J. Infect. Dis. 163*:47–52.

177. Okochi, K., Sato, H., Hinuma, Y. (1984). A retrospective study on transmission of adult T cell leukemia virus by blood transfusion: seroconversion in recipients. *Vox Sang. 46*:245–253.

178. Olafsson, K., Smith, M. S., Marshburn, P., Carter, S. G., Haskill, S. (1991). Variation of HIV infectibility of macrophages as a function of donor, stage of differentiation, and site of origin. *J. Acquir. Immune Defic. Syndr. 4*:154–164.

179. Osame, M., Matsumoto, M, Usuku, K. et al. (1987). Chronic progressive myelopathy associated with elevated antibodies to human T-lymphotropic virus type I and adult T-cell leukemia like cells. *Ann. Neurol. 21*:117–122.

180. Osame, M., Usuku, K., Izumo, S. et al. (1986). HTLV-I associated myelopathy, a new clinical entity. *Lancet 1*:1031–1032.

181. Ou, C. Y., Takebe, Y., Weniger, B. G., et al. (1993). Independent introduction of two major HIV-1 genotypes into distinct high-risk populations in Thailand. *Lancet 341*:1171–1174.

182. Padian, N., Marquis, L., Francis, D. P., et al. (1987). Male-to-female transmission of human immunodeficiency virus. *J. Am. Med. Assoc. 258*:788–790.

183. Pan, L. Z., Sheppard, H. W., Winkelstein, W., Levy, J. A. (1991). Lack of detection of human immunodeficiency virus in persistently seronegative homosexual men with high or medium risks for infection. *J. Infect. Dis. 164*:962–964.

184. Pantaleo, G., Graziosi, C., Demarest, J. F., et al. (1993). HIV infection is active and progressive in lymphoid tissue during the clinically latent stage of disease. *Nature 362*:355–358.

185. Pantaleo, G., Graziosi, C., Fauci, A. S. (1993). The immunopathogenesis of human immunodeficiency virus infection. *N. Engl. J. Med. 328*:327–335.

186. Pate, E. J., Wiktor, S. Z., Murphy, E., Champagnie, E., Ramlal, A., Blattner, W. A. (1995). Maternal-infant transmission of HTLV-I in Jamaica. Submitted.

187. Pezzotti, P., Rezza, G., Lazzarin, A., et al. (1992). Influence of gender, age, and transmission category on the progression from HIV seroconversion to AIDS. *J. Acquir. Immune Defic. Syndr. 5*:745–747.

188. Phillips, A. N., Lee C. A., Elford, J., Janossy, G., Kernoff, P. B. A. (1992). The cumulative risk of AIDS as the CD4 lymphocyte count declines. *J. Acquir. Immune Defic. Syndr. 5*:148–152.

189. Phillips, A. N., Lee, C. A., Elford, J. et al. (1991). More rapid progression to AIDS in older HIV-infected people: the role of CD4+ T-cell counts. *J. Acquir. Immune Defic. Syndr. 4*:970–975.

190. Piatak, M., Jr., Luk, K. C., Saag, M. S., et al. (1993). Viral dynamics in primary HIV-1 infection. *Lancet 341*:1099.

191. Piot, P., Laga, M., Ryder, R., et al. (1990). The global epidemiology of HIV infection: continuity, heterogeneity, and change. *J. Acquir. Immune Defic. Syndr. 3*:403–412.

192. Pluda, J. M., Venzon, D. J., Tosato, G., et al. (1993). Parameters affecting the development of non-Hodgkin's lymphoma in patients with severe human immunodeficiency virus infection receiving antiretroviral therapy. *J. Clin. Oncol. 11*:1099–1107.

193. Pluda, J. M., Yarchoan, R., Jaffe, E. S., et al. (1990). Development of non-Hodgkin lymphoma in a cohort of patients with severe human immunodeficiency virus

(HIV) infection on long-term antiretroviral therapy. *Ann. Intern. Med.* *113*:276–282.

194. Plummer, F. A., Simonsen, J. N., Ngugi, E. N., Cameron, D. W., Piot, P., Ndinya-Achola, J. O. (1985). Incidence of human immunodeficiency virus (HIV) infection and related disease in a cohort of Nairobi prostitutes. *Hepat. Scient.* M8.4.:6 abs.

195. Poiesz, B. J., Rusecetti, F. W., Gazdar, A. F., Bunn, P. A., Minna, J. D., Gallo, R. C. (1980). Detection and isolation of type-C retrovirus particles from fresh and cultured lymphocytes of a patient with cutaneous T-cell lymphoma. *Proc. Natl. Acad. Sci. USA 77*:7415–7419.

196. Pokrovsky, V. V., Kuznetsova, I., Eramova, I. (1990). Transmission of HIV-infection from an infected infant to his mother by breast-feeding. *Int. Conf. AIDS 6*:145.

197. Popovic, M, Gartner, S. (1987). Isolation of HIV-I from monocytes but not T-lymphocytes. *Lancet 2*:916.

198. Popovic, M., Sarngadharan, M.G., Read, E., Gallo, R.C. (1984). Detection, isolation, and continuous production of cytopathic retroviruses (HTLV–III) from patients with AIDS and pre-AIDS. *Science 224*:497–500

199. Potts, B. J., Maury, W., Martin, M. A. (1990). Replication of HIV-1 in primary monocyte cultures. *Virology 175*:465–476.

200. Reeves, W. C., Levine, P. H., Cuevas, M., Quiroz, E., Maloney, E., Saxinger, C. W. (1990). Seroepidemiology of human T-cell lymphotropic virus in the Republic of Panama. *Am. J. Trop. Med. Hyg. 42*:374–379.

201. Roberts, B. D., Foung, S. K. H., Lipka, J. J. et al. (1993). Evaluation of an immunoblot assay for serological confirmation and differentiation of human T-cell lymphotropic virus types I and II. *J. Clin. Microbiol. 31*:260–264.

202. Rosenberg, P. S., Gail, M. H., Carroll, R. J. (1992). Estimating HIV prevalence and projecting AIDS incidence in the United States: a model that accounts for therapy and changes in the surveillance definition of AIDS. *Stat. Med. 11*:1633–1655.

203. Rosenberg, P. S., Gail, M. H., Schrager, L. K., et al. (1991). National AIDS incidence trends and the extent of zidovudine therapy in selected demographic and transmission groups. *J. Acquir. Immune Defic. Syndr. 4*:392–401.

204. Rosenberg, P. S., Goedert, J. J., Biggar, R. J. (1994). Effect of age at seroconversion on the natural AIDS incubation distribution. *AIDS 8*:803–810.

205. Rosenblatt, J. D., Golde, D. W., Wachsman, W., et al. (1986). A second isolate of HTLV-II associated with atypical hairy cell leukemia. *N. Engl. J. Med. 315*:372–377.

206. Rosenblatt, J. D., Plaeger-Marshall, S., Giorgi, J. V., et al. (1990). A clinical, hemotologic, and immunologic analysis of 21 HTLV-II infected intravenous drug users. *Blood 76*:409–417.

207. Rossi, P., Moschese, V., Borliden, P. A., et al. (1989). Presence of maternal antibodies to human immunodeficiency virus 1 envelope glycoprotein gp120 epitopes correlates with the uninfected status of children born to seropositive mothers. *Proc. Natl. Acad. Sci. USA 86*:8055–8058.

208. Rous, P. (1911). A sarcoma of the fowl transmissible by an agent separable from the tumor cells. *J. Exp. Med. 13*:397.

209. Rubsamen-Waigmann, H., Briesen, H. V., Maniar, J. K., Rao, P. K., Scholz, C., Pfutzner, A. (1991). Spread of HIV-2 in India. *Lancet 337*:550–551.

210. Rudin, C., Berger, R., Tobler, R., Nars, P. W., Just, M., Pavic, N. (1990). HIV-1, hepatitis (A, B, and C), and measles in Romanian children. *Lancet 336*:1592–1593.

211. Saito, S., Ando, Y., Furuki, K., et al. (1990). Polymerase chain reaction (PCR) HTLV-I provirus detection of HTLV-I genome in infants born to HTLV-I seropositive mothers by polymerase chain reaction. *Acta Obset. Gynaec. Japan 42*:234–240.(abstract)

212. Samuel, M. C., Hessol, N., Shiboski, S., Engel, R. R., Speed, T. P., Windelstein, W., Jr. (1993). Factors associated with human immunodeficiency virus seroconversion in homosexual men in three San Francisco cohort studies, 1984–1989. *J. Acquir. Immune Defic. Syndr. 6*:303–312.

213. Sawanpanyalert, P., Ungchusak, K., Thanprasertsuk, S., Akarasewi, P. (1991). Seroconversion rate and risk factors for HIV-1 infection among low-class female sex workers in Chiangmai, Thailand: a multi cross-sectional study. *Seventh Int. Conf. AIDS*; WC3097.

214. Schneider, A. M., Straus, D. J., Schluger, A. E., et al. (1990). Treatment results with an aggressive chemotherapeutic regimen (MACOP-B) for intermediate-and some high-grade non-Hodgkins' lymphomas. *J. Clin. Oncol. 8*:94–102.

215. Schnittman, S. M., Greenhouse, J. J., Psallidopoulos, M. C., et al. (1990). Increasing viral burden in CD4+ T cells from patients with human immunodeficiency virus (HIV) infection reflects rapidly progressive immunosuppression and clinical disease. *Ann. Intern. Med. 113*:438–443.

216. Selik, R. M., Chu, S. Y., Buehler, J. W. (1993). HIV infection as leading cause of death among young adults in US cities and States. *J. Am. Med. Assoc. 269*:2991–2994.

217. Sharkey, S. J., Sharkey, K. A., Sutherland, L. R., Church, D. L. (1992). Nutritional status and food intake in human immunodeficiency virus infection. *J. Acquir. Immune Defic. Syndr. 5*:1091–1098.

218. Sheppard, H. W., Archer, M. S. (1991). AIDS and programmed cell death. *Immunol. Today 12*:423.

219. Sheppard, H. W., Ascher, M. S. (1992). The relationship between AIDS and immunologic tolerance. *J. Acquir. Immune Defic. Syndr. 5*:143–147.

220. Sheppard, H. W., Ascher, M. S., McRae, B., Anderson, R. E., Lang, W., Allain, J. (1991). The initial immune response to HIV and immune system activation determine the outcome of HIV disease. *J. Acquir. Immune Defic. Syndr. 4*:704–712.

221. Sherman, M. P., Dube, S., Spicer, T. P. et al. (1993). Sequence analysis of an immunogenic and neutralizing domain of the human T-cell lymphoma/leukemia virus type I gp46 surface membrane protein among various primate T-cell lymphoma/leukemia virus isolates including those from a patient with both human T-cell lym-

phoma/leukemia virus type I-associated myelopathy and adult T-cell leukemia. *Cancer Res. 53*:6067–6073.

222. Sherman, M. P., Saksena, N. K., Dube, D. K., Yanagihara, R., Poiesz, B. J. (1992). Evolutionary insights on the origin of human T-cell lymphoma/leukemia virus type I (HTLV-I) derived from sequence analysis of a new HTLV-I variant from Papua New Guinea. *J. Virol. 66*:2556–2563.

223. Shioiri, S., Tachibana, N., Okayama, A., et al. (1993). Analysis of anti-tax antibody of HTLV-I carriers in an endemic area in Japan. *Int. J. Cancer 53*:1–4.

224. Shiramizu, B., Herndier, B., McGrath, M. S. (1994). Identification of a common clonal human immunodeficiency virus integration site in human immunodeficiency virus-associated lymphomas. *Cancer Res. 54*:2069–2072.

225. Sidi, Y., Meytes, D., Shohat, B., et al. (1990). Adult T-cell lymphoma in Israeli patients of Iranian origin. *Cancer 65*:590–593.

226. Simonsen, J. N., Plummer, F. A., Ngugi, E. N., et al. (1990). HIV infection among lower socioeconomic strata prostitutes in Nairobi. *AIDS 4*:139–144.

227. Siraprapasiri, T., Thanprasertsuk, S., Rodklay, A. (1991). Risk factors for HIV among prostitutes in Chiangmai, Thailand. *AIDS 5*:579–582.

228. Sittitrai, W. (1990). Multi-stage interventions for sex workers in Thailand. *Proc. AIDS Asia Pacific Conf.* 165–171.

229. Sittitrai, W., Brown, T., Phanuphak, P., Barry, J., Sabaiying, M. (1991). The survey of partner relations and risk of HIV infection in Thailand. *Seventh Int. Conf. AIDS* MD 4113. (abstract)

230. Sommerfelt, M. A., Williams, B. P., Clapham, P. R., Solomon, E., Goodfellow, P. N., Weiss, R. A. (1988). Human T-cell leukemia viruses use a receptor determined by human chromosome 17. *Science 242*:1557–1559.

231. Spira, T. J., Kaplan, J. E., Feorino, P. M., Warfield, D. T., Fishbein, D. B., Bozeman, L. H. (1987). Human immunodeficiency virus viremia as a prognostic indicator in homosexual men with lymphadenopathy syndrome. *N. Engl. J. Med. 317*:1093–1094.

232. St. Louis, M. E., Kamenga, M., Brown, C., et al. (1993). Risk of HIV-1 transmission according to maternal immunologic, virologic, and placental factors. *J. Am. Med. Assoc. 269*:2853–2859.

233. Sullivan, M. T., Williams, A. E., Fang, C. T., Grandinetti, T., Poiesz, B. J., Ehrlich, G. D. (1991). Transmission of human T-lymphotropic virus type I and II by blood transfusion: a retrospective study of recipients of blood components (1983 through 1988). *Arch. Intern. Med. 151*:2043–2048.

234. Tachibana, N., Okayama, A., Ishihara, S., et al. (1992). High HTLV–I proviral DNA level associated with abnormal lymphocytes in peripheral blood from asymptomatic carriers. *Int. J. Cancer 51*:593–595.

235. Tachibana, N., Okayama, A., Ishizaki, J., et al. (1988). Suppression of tuberculin skin reaction in healthy HTLV-I carriers from Japan. *Int. J. Cancer 42*:829–831.

236. Tajima, K., Ito, S. I., Tsushima, A. T. L. Study Group (1990). Prospective Studies of HTLV-I and Associated Diseases in Japan. In Blattner, W. A., ed. *Human Retrovirology: HTLV.* New York: Raven Press, 267–279.

237. Tajima, K., Kamura, S., Ito, S., et al. (1987). Epidemiological features of HTLV-I carriers and incidence of ATL in an ATL-endemic island: A report of the community-based co-operative study in Tsushima, Japan. *Int. J. Cancer 40*:741–746.

238. Tajima, K. (1990). The T- and B-cell malignancy study group and co-authors. The 4th nation-wide study of adult T-cell leukemia/lymphoma (ATL) in Japan:estimates of risk of ATL and its geographical and clinical features. *Int. J. Cancer 45*:237–243.

239. Takatsuki, K., Uchiyama, T., Sagawa, K., Yodoi, J. (1976). Adult T-cell leukemia in Japan. In Seno, S., Takaku, F., Irino, S., eds. *Topics in Hematology*. Amsterdam: Excerpta Medica Amsterdam, 73–78.

240. Temin, H. M., Mizutani, S. (1970). RNA-dependent DNA polymerase in virions of Rous sarcoma virus. *Nature 226*:1211–1213.

241. Thompson, C. (1993). A slippery defence against HIV. *Lancet 342*:1500.

242. Tovo, P. A., De Martino, M., Gabiano, C. et al. (1992). Prognostic factors and survival in children with perinatal HIV-1 infection. *Lancet 339*:1249–1253.

243. Turner, B. J., Denison, M, Eppes, S. C., Houchens, R., Fanning, T., Markson, L. E. (1993). Survival experience of 789 children with acquired immunodeficiency syndrome. *Pediatr. Infect. Dis. J. 12*:310–320.

244. Uchiyama, T., Yodoi, J., Sagawa, K., Takatsuki, K., Uchino, H. (1977). Adult T-cell leukemia: Clinical and hematologic features of 16 cases. *Blood 50*:481–492.

245. Ungphakorn, J. (1990). The impact of AIDS on women in Thailand. *Proc. AIDS Asia Pacific Conf.* 151–154.

246. Van Griensvan, G. J. P., Samuel, M. C., Winkelstein, W., Jr. (1993). The success and failure of condom use by homosexual men in San Francisco. *J. Acquir. Immune Defic. Syndr. 6*:430–431.

247. Vanichseni, S., Choopanya, K., Des Jarlais, D. C., et al. (1992). HIV testing and sexual behavior among intravenous drug users in Bangkok, Thailand. *J. Acquir. Immune Defic. Syndr. 5*:1119–1123.

248. Varmus, H. (1988). Retroviruses. *Science 240*:1427–1435.

249. Wang, R. Y. H., Shih, J. W. K., Grandinetti, T., et al. (1992). High frequency of antibodies to mycoplasma penetrans in HIV-infected patients. *Lancet 340*:1312–1316.

250. Wawer, M. J., Serwadda, D., Musgrave, S. D., Konde-Lule, J. K., Musagara, M., Sewankambo, N. K. (1991). Dynamics of spread of HIV-1 infection in a rural district of Uganda. *Br. Med. J. 303*:1303–1306.

251. Wiktor, S. Z., Alexander, S. S., Shaw, G. M., et al. (1990). Distinguishing between HTLV-I and HTLV-II by Western blot. [Letter]. *Lancet 335*:1533.

252. Wiktor, S. Z., Pate, E. J., Murphy, E. L., et al. (1993). Mother-to-child transmission of human T-cell lymphotropic virus type I (HTLV-I) in Jamaica: association with antibodies to envelope glycoprotein (gp46) epitopes. *J. Acquir. Immune Defic. Syndr. 6*:1162–1167.

253. Williams, A. E., Fang, C. T., Slamon, D. J., et al. (1988). Seroprevalence and epidemiological correlates of HTLV-I infection in U.S. blood donors. *Science 240*:643–646.

254. Wolinsky, S. M., Wike, C. M., Korber, B. T. M., et al. (1992). Selective transmission of human immunodeficiency virus type-1 variants from mothers to infants. *Science* 255:1134–1137.

255. Wood, C. C., Williams, A. E., McNamara, J. G., Annunziata, J. A., Feorino, P. M., Conway, C. O. (1986). Antibody against the human immunodeficiency virus in commercial intravenous gammaglobulin preparations. *Ann. Intern. Med.* 105: 536–538.

256. Yamaguchi, K., Seiki, M., Yoshida, M, Nishimura, H., Kawano, F., Takatsuki, K. (1984). The detection of human T cell leukemia virus proviral DNA and its application for classification and diagnosis of T cell malignancy. *Blood* 63:1235–1240.

257. Yanagihara, R. (1992). Human T-cell lymphotropic virus type I infection and disease in the Pacific Basin. *Hum. Biol.* 64:843–854.

258. Yanagihara, R., Ajdukiewicz, A. B., Garruto, R. M., et al. (1991). Human T-lymphotropic virus type I infection in the Solomon Islands. *Am. J. Trop. Med. Hyg.* 44:122–130.

259. Yanagihara, R., Jenkins, C. L., Ajdukiewicz, A. B., Lal, R. B. (1991). Serological discrimination of HTLV-I and II infection in Melanesia. *Lancet* 337:617–618.

260. Yanagihara, R., Nerurkar, V. R. Garruto, R. M., et al. (1991). Characterization of a variant of human T-lymphotropic virus type I isolated from a healthy member of a remote, recently contacted group in Papua New Guinea. *Proc. Natl. Acad. Sci. USA* 88:1446–1450.

261. Zamora, T., Zaninovic, V., Kajiwara, M., Komoda, H., Hayami, M., Tajima, K. (1990). Antibody to HTLV-I in indigenous inhabitants of the Andes and Amazon regions in Colombia. *Japan J. Cancer Res.* 81:715–719.

262. Zaninovic, V., Zamora, T., Tajima, K. (1990). Origins of T-cell leukemia virus. *Nature* 344:299.

4

Viral protein targets of the immune response to varicella-zoster virus (VZV)

Ann M. Arvin
Stanford University School of Medicine
Stanford, CA 94305, USA

Varicella-zoster virus (VZV) causes varicella, commonly referred to as chicken pox, as a result of primary infection in susceptible individuals. The pathogenesis of primary infections includes a phase of initial viral replication after inoculation of respiratory mucosa followed by cell-associated viremia during which the virus is transported to skin sites. VZV viremia is much less intense than measles viremia; from 1:10,000 to 1:100,000 peripheral blood cells can be shown to harbor the virus by in situ hybridization (1). The intensity of the viremia corresponds to the severity of the rash, measured as the number of cutaneous vesicular lesions observed in healthy children. The viremic phase of primary VZV infection appears to be modulated by the cell-mediated immune response. Early studies of T–cell immunity to VZV, assessed by antigen-specific proliferation to VZV infected cell proteins in vitro, demonstrated that the interval to the detection of T–cells that recognize VZV correlated with how many lesions the child developed (2). Children who had an extensive rash usually lacked T–cell immunity when tested within the first 72 hours after the appearance of the first lesions. T–cell proliferation to VZV antigens was detected within 24–72 hours among children who had a minimal number of lesions. In addition, we observed that immune adults who were re-exposed to the virus, as mothers are while caring for children with varicella, showed a boost in their virus-specific T–cell proliferation

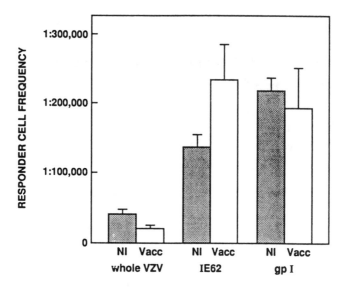

Figure 1 Responder cell frequencies of T–lymphocytes specific for the varicella-zoster virus whole antigen, immediate early protein (IE62), and gp I in
healthy adults with vaccine-induced or natural immunity to VZV as determined
by limiting dilution proliferation assay.

Varicella-zoster virus (VZV) specific responder cell frequencies ± standard
error (vertical axis) to whole VZV antigen, IE62 and gp I are shown in relation
to whether VZV immunity was naturally acquired (NI), indicated by the shaded
bars, or induced by immunization with varicella vaccine (vacc), indicated by
the open bars, as shown on the horizontal axis. Five subjects were tested in
each group.

Reprinted with permission (8).

(3). Immune adults with close contact with varicella cases did not develop
any signs of re-infection, but appeared to experience a subclinical re-
stimulation with VZV antigens in vivo. Herpes zoster is the second clinical illness that is caused by VZV. Herpes zoster is a consequence of the
fact that the virus establishes latency in cells of dorsal root ganglia following primary VZV infection. The virus can then reactivate to cause a
vesicular rash involving the dermatomal distribution of sensory nerves.
Susceptibility to VZV reactivation has been correlated with diminished
T–cell immunity in immunocompromised patients and in elderly people

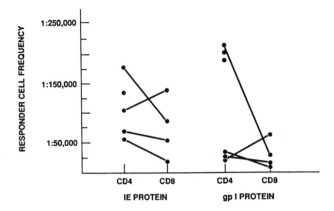

Figure 2   Precursor frequencies of cytotoxic T–lymphocytes specific for the immediate early (IE62) and glycoprotein I (gp I) of varicella-zoster virus within the CD4+ and CD8+ T–lymphocyte populations.

CD4+ and CD8+ T–lymphocyte populations were separated from peripheral blood by FACS under sterile conditions and incubated with inactivated VZV antigen in limiting dilution cultures; the initial T–cell concentrations ranged from 0, 1 x 10^3, 2 x 10^3, 1 x 10^4, 5 x 10^4 and 1 x 10^5. After 12 days, the effector cells were tested for lysis of autologous LCL infected with a vaccinia virus recombinant that expressed the VZV IE62 protein or gp I protein, or with a vaccinia control recombinant. Precursor frequency estimates were derived by statistical analysis of standard limiting dilution plots. T–lymphocytes from one donor was tested for CTL activity against the IE62 protein only and cells from two donors were tested with the gp I target only. T–cell subpopulations from four donors were evaluated against VZV IE62 protein or gp I targets in parallel; the points connected by lines indicate the precursor CTL frequencies from these assays.

Reprinted with permission (10).

(Review: 4). Episodes of VZV reactivation, in contrast to those caused by the related alpha herpes virus, herpes simplex virus, involve an extensive inflammatory response and cytopathic changes in the dorsal ganglia cell.

Our recent work has focused on identifying major VZV proteins that are recognized by human T–cells. These experiments have examined the host response to several of the VZV glycoproteins that are made abundantly in infected cells and constitute envelope proteins of the virus (5–8). We have also investigated the major regulatory protein of VZV,

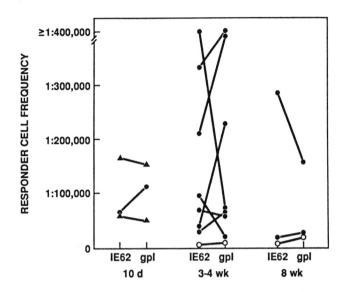

Figure 3   Kinetics of acquisition of cytotoxic T–lymphocytes specific for the varicella-zoster virus immediate early protein (IE62) and gp I following immunization with varicella vaccine.

VZV specific cytotoxic T–lymphocyte (CTL) frequency estimates (vertical axis) are shown for individual subjects who tested after one dose of varicella vaccine at intervals as indicated on the horizontal axis. Closed circles (0) indicate CTL frequencies for ten susceptible vaccine recipients; data for two vaccines who had pre-existing naturally acquired VZV immunity is shown with open circles (0). CTL frequencies in two subjects with recent acute varicella are indicated by triangles (Δ). The points connected by lines indicate CTL frequencies for IE62 and gp I targets as determined in the same subject.

Reprinted with permission (10).

which is called the immediate early (IE)–62 protein. In addition to its role as the major transactivating gene product, the IE–62 protein is a major component of the virion tegument (7). As a result, as soon as the virus enters the cell and is uncoated, the IE–62 protein becomes accessible to antigen processing and presentation systems, and could provide an early signal to the host that the cell is infected. We have also examined the role of the major DNA binding protein of VZV which is the product of

Table 1.1   *Varicella-zoster virus proteins and peptides recognized by T–lymphocytes from immune individuals*

Assay	T–cell subset	Viral protein
T–cell proliferation		
Proteins		gp I, gp II, gp III, pg IV, IE62
Peptides		gp I, gp II, gp IV, IE62
T–cell cytotoxicity		
Induction of clonal expansion by secondary stimulation	CD4+	gp I, gp II, gp IV
Recognition of target cells expressing VZV proteins	CD4+	gp I, gp IV, gp V, IE62
	CD8+	gp I, gp IV, gp V, IE62

Reprinted with permission (4).

ORF29 and is involved in viral replication. Initial studies of T–cell recognition of VZV proteins were done by using immunoaffinity purified glycoprotein I (gp I) or the IE–62 protein to stimulate T–cells in the proliferation assay (5,6,8). These experiments demonstrated that individuals with natural immunity to VZV maintain T–cells that recognize both of these proteins for many years after primary infection with the virus. In terms of responder cell frequencies, the immediate early gene product was recognized by approximately 1:100,000 T–cells and gp I was the target of about 1:200,000. The specificity of T–cell recognition of the IE–62 protein and gp I was further investigated by using the known amino acid sequences of each protein to select regions for preparation of synthetic peptides (9). Ten IE–62 and ten gp I peptides were made and used in the proliferation assay to determine what percentage of VZV immune donors from an "outbred" human population had T–cells that would recognize these peptides. Testing the panel of ten IE–62 peptides showed that most of these peptides were recognized by the majority of individuals. Similarly, when T–cells were stimulated with the gp I peptides, more than 60–70% of individuals had T–cell responses to most of the ten peptides.

A combination of two or three of the IE–62 and gp I peptides could be identified that were recognized by T–cells from all subjects who were evaluated, despite their diverse HLA phenotypes. In summary, in terms of proliferation responses to VZV proteins, our studies have shown that T–cell recognition of the IE–62 protein and glycoproteins I and III, is present immediately after primary infection and that it persists for at least twenty years after primary VZV infection.

In subsequent experiments, we examined the cytotoxic T–cell (CTL) response to IE–62 protein and the VZV glycoproteins, gp I, IV and V, to determine whether the proteins that elicit T–cell proliferation were also good targets for CTL recognition and whether the CTL response was characterized by any preferential recognition of specific VZV proteins. We have also evaluated the product of ORF29, the major DNA binding protein of VZV as a CTL target. These experiments were done in short-term limiting dilution cultures, using autologous EBV-transformed B cells super-infected with vaccinia recombinants expressing the VZV protein, as matched target cells. The EBV-transformed B cells express the VZV proteins abundantly when infected with VZV-vaccinia recombinants. The limiting dilution cytotoxicity assay provides data to define the responder cell frequencies for circulating T–lymphocytes that recognize a particular viral protein. Using this method, the numbers of memory T cells with specificity for IE–62 protein and gp I were equivalent, despite the fact that one is a major tegument/regulatory protein and the other is an envelope glycoprotein (10). When recognition of the intact IE–62 protein was compared to responses to a truncated form, which produces a fragment of only about 25% of the intact protein, again in the cytotoxicity assay, specific lysis was preserved at comparable levels. These experiments confirm that there are multiple regions of the IE–62 protein that can act as effective targets in the CTL response. The responder cell frequencies for CTL recognition of gp IV and gp V were in the same range, of approximately 1:100,000 as the IE–62 protein response, suggesting that all of these glycoproteins constitute good targets for T–cell recognition. In contrast, our recent experiments evaluating the ORF29 product which is made only in infected cells during active replication, is not as good a target for cytotoxicity as the IE–62 protein or the glycoproteins.

Another issue that we have addressed in the analysis of T–cell mediated cytotoxicity in VZV immunity was to determine the phenotype of the predominant cytotoxic effector cells in the short term limiting dilution assay (10). These experiments were performed using fresh peripheral blood mononuclear cells, separating the cells by flow cytometry to generate two CD4+ and CD8+ populations that were more than 99% pure, and incubating each T–cell population with VZV antigen and autologous antigen-presenting cells. These experiments demonstrated that the numbers of effector T–cells specific for VZV IE–62 protein and gp I in either the CD4 and CD8 populations was equivalent, based upon statistical comparisons of parallel lysis using T–cells from twelve unrelated donors.

The clinical experience in immunocompromised individuals who have had past infection with VZV, and are therefore latently infected with the virus, demonstrates the significance of the T–cell immune response. Bone marrow transplant recipients represent a population at high risk for VZV reactivation, causing herpes zoster, which is extensive in the primary dermatome and visceral dissemination of the virus due to cell-associated viremia. When the responder cell frequencies specific for VZV were enumerated in bone marrow transplant patients in comparison with normal, healthy immune subjects, CTL frequencies for both the IE protein and the gp 1 protein were markedly diminished (11). Analysing the T–cell subsets present in the limiting dilution cultures demonstrated that the bone marrow transplant patients had many fewer CD4+ T–cells after incubation with VZV antigen than naturally immune subjects; the numbers of CD8+ T–cells were approximately the same for immunocompromised and healthy subjects. When the bone marrow transplant recipients were evaluated late after transplantation, it was possible to demonstrate the recovery of T–cell responses to VZV in many patients. Reconstitution of immunity could be attributed to clinically symptomatic reactivation of the the virus, causing herpes zoster in some patients, but in others, we demonstrated that subclinical reactivations may also function to restore VZV specific responses. Using polymerase chain reaction to detect virus in peripheral blood mononuclear cells, we found that a significant percentage of asymptomatic patients had evidence of subclinical VZV infection; 17% of bone marrow transplant recipients who were studied during the first 6 months after transplantation had VZV viremia by PCR (11).

VZV is the first human herpes virus for which licensure of a live, atte-nuated vaccine is anticipated. In another series of experiments, we have examined the T–cell response in healthy susceptible individuals who have been immunized with the investigational, live attenuated varicella vaccine, the Oka/Merck vaccine (6,8,12,13). Initial studies of the T–cell proliferation response to the IE–62 protein and gp I showed that individu-als given the Oka/Merck vaccine who were tested at six weeks and one year after immunization, had circulating memory T–cells that recognized both of these proteins (6,8). An analysis of the kinetics of the appearance of CTLs that recognized the IE–62 protein and gp I showed effective cy-totoxicity from 10 days to 3–4 weeks after vaccination. When two indi-viduals who were already immune to VZV were given the vaccine, a very marked increase in CTL frequencies, to 1:5000–1:10,000 cells was ob-served. This finding about CTL enhancement is important because it con-firms the evidence from T–cell proliferation assays that the varicella vaccine may be useful to increase T–cell recognition in elderly individu-als who are at risk for VZV reactivation as herpes zoster. When the kinet-ics of the initial response within the CD4+ and the CD8+ populations was examined, whether the initial response was to IE–62 protein or gp I and whether it was mediated predominantly by CD4+ or CD8 T–cells was variable, however, vaccines developed CTL in both subsets that recog-nized both proteins within 8–12 weeks (13). Immunization with the live attenuated varicella vaccine also elicited T–cells that recognized gp IV and gp V. The response to gp V was more variable among individual vac-cinees, which may be due to diminished production of this protein by Oka strain.

Finally, we have evaluated the capacity of individual VZV proteins to elicit T–cell responses when given as primary immunogens in the guinea pig model of VZV (14–16). Immunization with the glycoproteins, gp I, IV or V, or with the IE–62 protein expressed in vaccinia recombinants re-sulted in detectable T–cell proliferation to VZV antigens. When the ani-mals were challenged with infectious VZV, a marked boost in T–cell responses to VZV antigen was elicited. In contrast, evidence of priming was not detected in animals immunized with the major DNA binding pro-tein (ORF29 product). When these animals were challenged with infec-tious virus, there was no protection against cell associated viremia in comparison to parallel cohorts of animals inoculated with vaccinia expressing the IE–62 protein.

In summary, T–cells that recognize the major VZV glycoproteins and the major immediate early tegument protein (ORF62) persist in individuals with both natural and vaccine-induced immunity. The memory T–cell response to the major DNA-binding protein (ORF29) is less predictable. Cytotoxic T–cell recognition exhibits no predominance for IE–62 protein as opposed to glycoprotein-expressing targets and CTL effector cells can be demonstrated in both the CD4+ and the CD8+ T–cell populations. Experiments in bone marrow transplant recipients indicate the need for persistent T–cell immunity to maintain VZV latency and that subclinical as well as symptomatic reactivations may restore virus specific immunity in these patients. Studies in the guinea pig model suggest that specific viral glycoproteins and the IE–62 protein may be effective immunogens in protection against primary VZV infection in vivo.

Acknowledgments

Vaccinia recombinants used in these experiments were provided by our collaborators, Drs. John Hay, William Rucheyan, Paul Kinchington and colleagues. The studies of VZV immunity were supported by the National Institute of Allergy and Infectious Diseases (AI20459 and AI22280) and by Merck & Co., Inc.

References

1. Koropchak, C. M., Solem, S., Diaz, P. S., Arvin, A. M. (1989). Investigation of varicella-zoster virus infection of lymphocytes by *in situ* hybridization. *J. Virol.* *63*:2392–2395.
2. Arvin A. M., Koropchak C. M., Williams B. R. G., Grumet, F. C. and Foung S. K. (1986). Early immune response in healthy and immunocompromised subjects with primary varicella-zoster virus infection. *J. Infect. Dis. 154*:422–9.
3. Arvin A. M., Koropchak, C. M., and Wittek, A. E. (1983). Immunologic evidence for re-infection with varicella-zoster virus. *J. Infect. Dis. 148*:200–205.
4. Arvin A. M. (1992). Cell-mediated immunity to varicella-zoster virus. *J. Infect. Dis. 166* Suppl 1:S35–41.

5. Arvin, A. M., Kinney-Thomas, E., Shriver, K. et al. (1986). Immunity to varicella-zoster viral glycoproteins, gp I (90/58) and gp III (gp 118) and to a nonglycosylated protein, p170. *J. Immunol. 137*:1346–1351.

6. Diaz P. S., Smith, S., Hunter, E., Arvin A. M. (1988). Immunity to varicella-zoster virus antigen, glycoprotein I (gp I) and a non-glycosylated protein (p. 170): relation to the immunizing regimen of live attenuated varicella vaccine. *J. Infect. Dis. 158*:1245–52.

7. Kinchington, P. R., Houghland, J. K., Arvin, A. M., Ruyechan, W. T., Hay, I. (1992). Varicella zoster virus IE62 protein is a major virion component. *J. Virol. 66*:359–66.

8. Bergen, R. E., Diaz, P. S., Arvin, A. M. (1990). The immunogenicity of the Oka/ Merck varicella vaccine in relation to infectious varicella-zoster virus and relative viral antigen content. *J. Infect. Dis. 162*:1049–54.

9. Bergen, R. E., Sharp, M., Sanchez, Judd A. K., Arvin, A. M. (1991). Diversity of human cell-mediated immune recognition of the immediate early protein, IE62, and the glycoprotein I of varicella-zoster virus. *Viral Immunol. 4*:151–66.

10. Arvin, A. M., Sharp, M. S., Smith, S. et al. (1991). Equivalent recognition of a varicella-zoster virus immediate early protein (IE62) and glycoprotein I by cytotoxic T–lymphocytes of either CD4+ or CD8+ phenotype. *J. Immunol. 146*:257–64.

11. Wilson, A., Sharp, M., Koropchak, C. M., Ting, S. F., Arvin, A. M. (1992). Subclinical varicella-zoster virus viremia, herpes zoster and recovery of T–lymphocyte responses to varicella-zoster viral antigens after allogeneic and autologous bone marrow transplantation. *J. Infect. Dis. 165*:119–26.

12. Diaz, P. D., Smith, S., Hunter, E., and Arvin, A. M. (1989). T–lymphocyte cytotoxicity with natural varicella-zoster virus infection and after immunization with live attenuated varicella vaccine. *J. Immunol. 142*:636–41.

13. Sharp, M., Terada, K., Wilson, A., Nader, S., Kinchington, P. E., Ruyechan, W., Hay, J., Arvin, A. M. (1992). The kinetics and protein specificity of T–lymphocyte cytotoxicity in healthy adults immunized with live attenuated varicella vaccine. *J. Infect. Dis. 165*:852–8.

14. Arvin, A. M., Solem, S. M., Koropchak, C. M., et al. (1987). Humoral and cellular immunity to varicella-zoster virus glycoprotein, gp I, and to a non-glycosylated protein, p 170, in the strain 2 guinea pig. *J. Gen. Virol. 68*:2449–2454.

15. Lowry, P. W., Solem, S., Watson, B. N., Koropchak, C. M., Kinchington, P. E., Ruyechan, W., Hay, J., Arvin, A. M. (1992). Immunity in strain 2 guinea pigs inoculated with vaccinia recombinants expressing varicella-zoster virus glycoproteins I, IV, V or the immediate early gene 62. *J. Gen. Virol. 73*:811–19.

16. Sabella, C., Lowry, P. W., Abbruzzi, G. M., Koropchak, C. M., Kinchington, P. R., Sadegh-Zadeh, M., Hay, J., Ruyechan, W. T., Arvin, A. M. (1993). Immunization with the immediate-early tegument protein (Open Reading Frame 62) of varicella-zoster virus protects guinea pigs against virus challenge. *J. Virol. 67*:7673–76.

5

Pathogenic aspects of measles virus infections

Sibylle Schneider-Schaulies, Jürgen Schneider-Schaulies,
Jens-Jörg Schnorr, and Volker ter Meulen
*Institute for Virology and Immunology, University of Würzburg,
Versbacher Str. 7, D–97078 Würzburg, Germany*

Martin A. Billeter
*Institute for Molecular Biology II Eidgenössische Technische
Hochschule Hönggerberg, CH–8093 Zürich, Switzerland*

Introduction

Infection of seronegative individuals with measles virus (MV) usually leads to acute measles, an epidemic disease with a world-wide prevalence. As a consequence of the successful application of a live vaccine, the incidence of acute measles has been significantly reduced in industrialized countries. In developing countries, however, this disease is still among the primary causes of infant death. Moreover, recent epidemiological studies in North America revealed that measles virus vaccination in early childhood does not provide life-long immunity since measles has also occurred there in prevaccinated children and young adults (Gustafson et al., 1987). Altogether, the high rate of MV-associated complications worldwide demands new measles research initiatives and is a challenge for the development of new measles vaccines and vaccination strategies. In the following paper MV-associated diseases and their pathogenesis will briefly be reviewed.

Diseases caused by measles virus

A well defined disease process is encountered in the case of acute measles. The virus is efficiently spread by aerosol and replicates first in the respiratory tract. Subsequently it reaches local lymphatic tissue. After amplification in lymph node tissue, a viremia leads to the dissemination of the virus to multiple lymphoid tissues and other organs including skin, liver and the gastrointestinal tract. The viremia is cell associated and MV can be detected in peripheral blood mononuclear cells (PBMCs), in particular in monocytes (Esolen et al., 1993). Besides the classical disease of acute measles which develops after an incubation period of approximately 10 days, the infection can also lead to modified or atypical measles depending on the patient's immune status. Modified measles develops in children exposed to measles who have received a gammaglobulin injection in an amount insufficient to abort the infection or in infants with transplacentally transmitted maternal measles antibodies. The incubation period is longer than in classical measles and the illness is shorter with much milder clinical symptoms. Atypical measles can develop in children who had received inactivated measles vaccine and are exposed later to wild measles virus. Atypical measles has a sudden onset with high fever, headache, pleural and abdominal pain. The rash has a distinct centripetal distribution and in some patients it is spotty, involving only the wrist and ankles. In addition, pneumonitis and pleuritis lead to severe illness. The pathogenesis of atypical measles is linked to the observation that immunization with killed measles vaccine does not lead to the development of sufficient antibodies against MV F protein (Norrby et al., 1975). Therefore, viral spread from cell to cell by cell fusion is not blocked. It is obvious that the development of any new measles vaccine including subunit vaccines have to take into account that partial immunity may lead to complications.

During acute measles, complications may arise which consist of diarrhea, pneumonia, laryngotracheobronchitis, otitis media and stomatitis. In developing countries, increased case fatality is associated with age of infection and nutritional status. Of particular clinical relevance is the development of acute measles encephalitis during or shortly after acute measles which occurs at a relatively constant rate throughout different populations in around 0.1% of cases. This complication has a mortality rate of 10–30%. This encephalitis is not the result of a direct virus invasion of the CNS, but rather the consequence of a measles virus induced autoimmune reaction against brain antigen (Moench et al., 1988) (see below).

In contrast, late complications associated with MV are rare. These are subacute sclerosing panencephalitis (SSPE) and, in immunocompromised individuals, measles inclusion body encephalitis (MIBE) (ter Meulen et al., 1983). These fatal diseases exhibit virological and immunological features quite different from those seen in acute measles or measles encephalitis. Both diseases develop on the basis of a persistent MV infection in brain cells. Giant cell formation and budding virus particles as typically found in measles infection, are virtually absent in SSPE or MIBE brain, indicating defective MV replication in CNS tissue. This is supported by the observation that MV cannot be isolated by standard isolation procedures, but only occasionally by cocultivation methods (see below).

Immunological changes pathognomonic for SSPE include exceptionally high antibody titers to the majority of measles virus structural proteins except the membrane (M) protein in serum and CSF specimens and a prominent immunoglobulin elevation in CSF. This latter finding specifically relates to an increase in IgG that exhibits restricted banding on electrophoresis indicating an MV-specific oligoclonal population of IgG. The occurrence of IgG elevation with measles-specific oligoclonal IgG in the CSF of these patients reflects a state of CNS hyperimmunization against this agent and results from a local production of antiviral antibodies by sensitized lymphocytes which have invaded this compartment (ter Meulen et al., 1983).

MIBE in general is rather similar to SSPE (Roos et al., 1981, Ohuchi et al., 1987), although there are some important differences. In comparison to SSPE, the incubation periods between acute measles and onset of MIBE are shorter and the clinical course is more of an acute nature. The most obvious difference, however, is that in MIBE no hyperimmune response to MV is mounted as the immune system is generally impaired due to other systemic diseases.

Diseases putatively associated with measles virus

Whereas MV has been etiologically linked to SSPE and MIBE, there are other well defined diseases in which there is some suggestive indirect evidence of an involvement of measles virus (Cosby, 1993). In particular, in multiple sclerosis (MS) MV is still among the candidate viruses as many MS patients exhibit a humoral hyperimmune response against MV antigens in serum and CSF specimens (ter Meulen and Stephenson, 1983) and MV-specific RNA has been located by *in situ* hybridization in some MS brains (Haase et al., 1981, Cosby et al., 1989). Similarly, a pathogenic role of MV has been suggested for Morbus Padget, a chronic progressive disorder of bones of unknown etiology and otosclerosis, a common cause of hearing loss in Caucasian adults (Basle et al., 1986, McKenna and Mills, 1989). In both diseases, MV 'footprints' were detected in bone lesions. However, these findings are unconfirmed and it remains to be elucidated whether MV is of pathogenetic importance or merely an opportunistic pathogen in these disorders. The last group of diseases which have been associated with measles virus are various autoimmune syndromes such as chronic hepatitis, glomerulonephritis and Lupus erythematodes (Robertson et al., 1987, Andjaparidze et al., 1989). In these disorders, either a humoral hyperimmune response is found against measles virus or MV RNA has been detected in peripheral lymphocytes of these patients. So far, no additional data exist which would indicate that measles virus plays a pathogenetic role in these diseases.

Measles virus gene expression in neural tissue

As indicated by the lack of infectious virus in brain material of patients with SSPE and MIBE, MV gene expression is expected to be restricted, however, allowing the virus to survive in a cell associated form inaccessible to the host immune surveillance. This is, in general, achieved by maintaining the expression of the viral protein functions essential for transcription and replication of the viral genome, and by reducing or abolishing the expression of the envelope proteins. Indeed, in most of the infected brain cells N and P proteins can be detected, whereas M, F and H proteins are, if at all, present only in low amounts in a small percentage of infected cells (Liebert et al., 1986). In order to define the basis for the re-

strictions observed, viral RNAs and their biological activity were analysed directly from brain material of patients with persistent CNS
infections. As a second source, virus isolates obtained by cocultivation of
SSPE brain material with permissive tissue culture cells were available.
For detailed analysis, cDNA clones containing the entire coding sequences or subgenic fragments of MV structural genes were sequenced
and expressed *in vitro* (reviewed by Billeter and Cattaneo, 1991; Schneider-Schaulies and ter Meulen, 1992).

Transcriptional attenuation of MV

One of the hallmarks of attenuated MV gene functions in persistent infections of the human CNS is the relatively low frequency of envelope gene
specific mRNAs. Whereas in lytically infected nonneural tissue culture
cells the H-specific transcript is expressed with a relative frequency of 20
to 30% compared to the N–mRNA, in SSPE brain material it is reduced to
about 1% (Cattaneo et al., 1987 a, b). This underrepresentation of the envelope gene specific mRNAs may well contribute to the low expression
of the corresponding proteins in brain tissue (Liebert et al., 1986). In
addition, qualitative alterations of MV transcription indicated by an increased frequency of bicistronic transcripts have been observed. In one
case of SSPE and a persistently infected cell line, the failure to detect M
protein could be linked to a complete replacement of the P and M mono-
cistronic mRNAs by a bicistronic transcript (Baczko et al. 1986, Cattaneo
et al., 1987b). As within the corresponding intergenic regions and their
flanking regions, no striking sequence alterations could be detected, the
reason for this particular transcriptional regulation still has to be determined.

Introduction of mutations into the MV genome

Point mutations

A reliable estimation of the frequency of mutations accumulating in MV
genes during the clinical inapparent incubation periods for MIBE and
SSPE has been hampered by the fact that the sequence of the infecting

wild type MV, is not available. Recent studies demonstrated that circulating wild type measles virus isolates can be subdivided into several strains differing overall in 1 to 2% of their nucleotide sequences (Taylor et al., 1991, Rota et al., 1992, Baczko et al., 1992). Thus, individual SSPE viruses resemble certain substrains to a much higher degree than anticipated previously based on comparison with a consensus sequence (Billeter and Cattaneo, 1991). However, on average still one percent of nucleotide differences are encountered between SSPE viruses and their closest known lytic relatives (Wong et al., 1991). Most mutations encountered are scattered point mutations introduced by polymerase errors. In general, each type of nucleotide transition is about ten times more frequent than each type of transversion. Silent mutations are equally distributed in the genome, whereas expressed mutations are most frequent in the M gene, and progressively lower in the P, N, H and F genes (Billeter and Cattaneo, 1991). The high mutability of the M gene in SSPE is striking in view of the general high conservation of the M genes in *Paramyxoviridae* (variability P > H = N > F = M > L, Rima, 1989).

Hypermutations

As a second type of mutation, simultaneous clustered transitions leading to an exchange of uridine (U) by cytidine (C) residues or, less frequent, adenosine (A) by guanosine (G) residues in the positive strand have been found, first in the MV M gene (Cattaneo et al., 1989). The most plausible explanation for this finding was provided by the action of a cellular unwindase activity converting up to 50% of A residues in synthetic double stranded RNAs into inosine (I) (Bass and Weintraub, 1987, Wagner and Nishikura, 1988). The unwindase, now referred to as duplex RNA dependent adenosine deaminase (DRADA), has been detected in extracts of a variety of eucaryotic tissue culture cells *in vitro*, unwinding and modifying double stranded RNAs without any obvious sequence specificity (Nishikura et al., 1991). Thus, extensive dsRNA structures as those occurring erroneously during transcription and replication of negative stranded RNA viruses may provide ideal target structures for the DRADA. The potential relevance of the DRADA for modulating gene functions of RNA viruses is supported by the fact that clustered hypermutations have been also observed for vesicular stomatitis virus (O'Hara et al., 1984), human parainfluenza 3 (Murphy et al., 1991) and bunyavirus (Antic et al., 1992). For MV, hypermutated sequences have been identified repeatedly in several independent cases of SSPE and MIBE, mainly located in the M gene (Cattaneo et al., 1989, Baczko et al., 1993). In tissue culture, hypermutated M- and, for the 1P3–Ca cell line, H-sequences have been isolated from SSPE derived viruses (for reviews see Billeter and Cattaneo, 1991, Billeter et al., 1994). Recent *in vitro* analyses confirmed the presence and high activity of the unwindase in nuclear and cytoplasmic extracts of human neural cells (Rataul et al., 1992, Ecker et al., 1995).

Distribution of mutations in the MV genes and their functional consequences

The genes of the viral core proteins N, P and probably L in SSPE viruses do not reveal any changes of their coding sequences suggestive of modifying gene functions, since the replicative potential of the virus has to be maintained. In contrast, profound alterations of the SSPE M genes resulting in a decreased stability (Sheppard et al., 1986), premature termination or complete inactivation of the corresponding proteins (Cattaneo et al., 1989) have been attributed to expressed mutations. Impairments of the M protein function are evident in these cases, but this may also result from less spectacular amino acid exchanges which lead to conformational changes of the protein as shown by Hirano and coworkers (1993). However, M gene sequence changes might not be a prerequisite for the development of SSPE since intact wildtype-like M reading frames have been found (Cattaneo et al., 1989, Baczko et al., 1993). On the other hand, a selective advantage for the virus spread in the CNS seems to be associated with the abrogation of M protein function since the prevalence of one of five mutated M sequences were found in different brain regions of one patient with SSPE (Baczko et al., 1993). This interpretation is supported by the finding that a virus isolated from an SSPE patient carrying a defective M gene dominantly interfered with the replication of wild type virus in a cell fusion assay in tissue culture (Hirano, 1992).

Another interesting observation is the mutations occurring at the cytoplasmic tail of the MV F proteins. In all SSPE cases studied, point mutations have led to a premature termination of the reading frame except for one case where the normal stop codon was abolished resulting in the elongation of the coding sequence (Schmid et al., 1992, Cattaneo and Rose, 1993, reviewed in Billeter et al., 1994). Interestingly, these typical alterations have not been encountered in MIBE cases so far.

The mutations found within the H genes have not been linked to alterations of the reading frames; some lead to the elimination or creation of glycosylation sites (Cattaneo and Rose, 1993). Moreover, addition of complex oligosaccharides and dimerisation required for an efficient cell surface transport have been found to be more or less affected for SSPE derived H proteins. Progress toward the definition of motifs essential for glycoprotein function has been made by using recombinant vaccinia virus based expression systems (Cattaneo and Rose, 1993). Most of the SSPE H proteins failed to exert their fusion helper function when coexpressed with heterologous F protein derived from the Edmonston vaccine strain indicating their functional impairment. However, coexpression with their homologous corresponding F proteins gave rise to extensive cell fusion suggesting that the mode of cooperation between both proteins in fusion activity which requires specific F–H interactions are apparently retained during persistence. Thus, MV genomes spread through the CNS probably may occur by localized cell fusion.

The establishment of persistent infections: primary interactions between MV and neural cells

As pointed out in the previous section, persistent infection in SSPE or MIBE at the time of death is characterised by defective viral genomes that are generally unable to undergo a productive replication cycle even when transferred to permissive cells. However, nothing is known about the events which lead to the establishment of persistent infection, when and how the virus enters the brain, which intracellular factors determine brain cell tropism and precisely how the virus spreads in the brain in the absence of infectious virus particles and documented cell fusion events. To study these aspects, we established an animal model and used tissue culture systems with primary and permanent cells of neural and non-neural origin.

The animal model

Following intracerebral inoculation of a neurotropic rat brain adapted CAM-strain of MV, inbred Lewis rats develop, after different incubation periods, an acute or subacute measles encephalomyelitis (Liebert and ter Meulen, 1987). Neuropathological findings in the acute encephalitis include focal mononuclear cell infiltration in the grey matter of both cerebral hemispheres and basal ganglia usually with little or no degenerative changes. Extensive perivascular infiltrations of mononuclear cells in the grey and white matter of the brain hemispheres, mid-brain and upper spinal cord is encountered in rats with clinical signs of subacute encephalitis (SAME). Extracellular virus particles and giant cell formation are not detectable. Infectious virus can only be isolated from rats with acute encephalitis but not from animals with SAME. Furthermore, already during the acute phase of infection and disease the expression of the envelope proteins M, F and H in infected brain cells is reduced. In SAME, this reduction is more pronounced, in some cases beyond the detection level, suggesting that similar factors are probably interfering with viral replication as observed in SSPE or MIBE. Indeed, analysis of MV-specific transcription in brain material isolated from Lewis rats with acute and subacute encephalitis revealed a restricted expression of the viral envelope proteins which was linked to an attenuated expression of the corresponding mRNAs (Schneider-Schaulies et al., 1989). In the case of SAME, a specific translational defect could be found for the M specific mRNA that was not related to sequence mutations (Schneider-Schaulies and ter Meulen, 1992). As these transcriptional alterations were observed in primary rat astroglial cells early in infection but not in Vero cells, host cell dependent control mechanisms of viral transcription were suggestive (Schneider-Schaulies et al., 1990). It should be kept in mind that SAME in rats differs in important aspects from SSPE in particular by its high incidence, the short time course and the artificial inoculation procedure.

Cellular factors controlling MV transcription and translation

In analyzing potential host factors it became obvious that spontaneous reduction of MV transcription was up to 10-fold reduced in human neural tissue culture cells compared to non-neural controls (Schneider-Schaulies et al., 1993). In addition, the differentiation state of the cells influence active transcription of MV as seen in brain material of experimentally infected animals (Liebert et al., 1990a) and in tissue culture upon *in vitro* differentiation of neuronal cells (Yoshikawa and Yamanouchi, 1984). Moreover, an enhanced attenuation of MV transcription was found in the presence of virus-neutralizing antibodies as a result of antibody-induced antigenic modulation (Schneider-Schaulies et al., 1992). Initial observations indicated that the exogenous application of anti-MV sera as well as virus-neutralising anti-H-antibodies led to the downregulation of intracellular MV protein synthesis in rat glioma and mouse neuroblastoma cells, but not in nonneural cells persistently infected with MV (Barrett et al., 1985, Rager-Zisman et al., 1984). In further studies, a general downregulation of MV transcription 24 hours after the application of neutralising antibodies was found without affecting the slope of the transcription gradient (Schneider-Schaulies et al., 1992). The signal transducing pathway, leading to an intracellular regulation of MV gene expression following the interaction of MV antibodies with a surface molecule on persistently infected neural cells, has not yet been defined. However, treatment of persistently infected rat glioma cells with measles antibodies led to a G protein-mediated induction of inositol polyphosphate production followed by the activation of protein kinase C (Weinmann-Dorsch et al., 1990). Although the relationship between this activation and the control of viral gene expression has not been established, alterations of cellular kinase activities may well be highly significant for the viral gene expression. In particular, phosphorylation of viral proteins present in the transcription complex might modulate the activity as suggested for the P proteins of VSV (Sleat et al., 1993).

Consistent with these findings was the observation that passive transfer of neutralizing anti-H antibodies to MV infected newborn Lewis rats had a pronounced effect on the disease course (Liebert et al., 1990b). Instead of acute necrotizing encephalopathy occurring in control animals within few days, in antibody treated animals a subacute encephalitis after a prolonged incubation period was established. In brain material of these animals, viral transcription proved to be highly attenuated at the single cell level accompanied by a very low frequency of the envelope specific mRNAs. A remarkably similar pattern was detected in brain material of experimentally infected BN rats naturally mounting high titers of virus-neutralising antibodies.

Although convincing evidence has been presented for the effect of sequence mutations on MV gene function in SSPE brain, they do not seem to be essential in the animal model, since the M gene specific mRNA in brain material of Lewis rats with SAME is impaired in the absence of mutations in the corresponding reading frame. Evidence for cellular mechanisms controlling MV gene expression on the translational level has been provided after *in vitro* differentiation of human glial cells (Schneider-Schaulies et al., 1993). Under these conditions, normal amounts of viral mRNAs were synthesized as compared to undifferentiated cells. These mRNAs were able to direct the synthesis of viral proteins *in vitro*, whereas viral protein synthesis in the infected cells was highly inefficient. This effect could not be observed using nonneural cells suggesting host cell specific regulatory components. These may include a specific response to external infection dependent stimuli such as interferons. In fact, it has been demonstrated that human MxA protein that is widely expressed after IFN-treatment of most tissue culture cells is only capable of interfering with MV primary transcription when expressed in human brain cells (Schneider-Schaulies et al., 1994). Whether or not this finding is relevant for the establishment of persistent MV CNS infections and what would be the mechanism underlying MxA-mediated restriction of MV transcription remains to be established.

Measles virus induced autoimmune reactions against brain antigen

Of particular pathogenetic interest is the development of measles encephalomyelitis as a complication of acute measles. Based on the absence of MV RNA and protein in CNS tissue together with the neuropathological changes, an immunopathological basis for the development of this CNS complication is suggestive. So far, this interpretation is only supported by circumstantial evidence. In patients with acute measles encephalomyelitis a significant proliferative response of isolated peripheral lymphocytes against myelin basic protein (MBP) was found, which was recorded not only during the clinical symptoms, but also as late as 30 days after the onset of disease (Johnson et al., 1984). Moreover, in CSF specimens from such patients, MBP protein was detected as a consequence of myelin breakdown. In addition to these cell mediated immune (CMI) responses to MBP, patients with MV encephalomyelitis reveal prolonged immuno-logical abnormalities, in particular elevation of IgE as well as lower titers of soluble IL–2 receptor in comparison to patients with uncomplicated measles (Griffin et al., 1985, 1989). Such MBP specific lymphoprolifera-tive responses have not only been seen after measles infection but also after postinfectious encephalomyelitis following rubella, varicella and re-spiratory infection and in patients with complications of postexposure ra-bies immunization (Johnson and Griffin, 1986). The latter disorder is probably the human equivalent of experimental allergic encephalomyeli-tis (EAE) since such patients received rabies vaccine prepared in brain tissue. By analogy to EAE it is not surprising, therefore, that the finding of MBP specific lymphoproliferative response in these virus infections is considered to be of pathogenetic importance.

Measles virus induced CMI responses to MBP in experimental animals

The available evidence of a possible immunopathological basis of measles encephalomyelitis demanded animal experiments to study in de-tail the mechanism by which a measles infection leads to these adverse immunological effects. In this context, the infection of Lewis rats with a neurotropic MV strain as described above is of interest since these ani-mals reveal neuropathological changes which resemble to some extent those of EAE.

It has been shown in EAE in Lewis rats that an autoimmune disease of the CNS can be induced by injection of MBP or proteolytic apoprotein in combination with Freund's complete adjuvants (Raine, 1984, Yamamura et al., 1986). This disease is characterized by transient clinical signs con-sisting of weak or paralysed hindlimbs and weight loss. Neuropathologically, inflammatory changes consisting mainly of perivascular cuffings is commonly found predominantly in the white matter of the spinal cord. In addition, spinal cord demyelination can be observed although its appearance depends to some extent on the inoculum used (Itoyama and Webster, 1982, Vandenbark et al., 1985). Moreover, EAE can be passively transferred from a diseased to a naive recipient animal with CD4+ lymphocytes specific for MBP. This treatment produces in the host animal a CNS disorder which is clinically and neuropathologically very similar to EAE (Raine, 1984)

In our rat model, infection with the neurotropic MV leads to the development of a subacute measles encephalomyelitis 4–8 weeks after infection. The CNS changes are very similar to those of donor rats receiving MBP specific CD4+ lymphocytes and splenic lymphocytes from these animals were found to proliferate *in vitro* in the presence of MBP (Liebert et al., 1988). MBP-specific class II MHC restricted T cell lines were isolated from these cell populations. They were shown to exhibit no crossreactivity with MV and to induce EAE in naive syngeneic recipients following adoptive transfer. The clinical and histopathological signs of this T cell mediated disease were identical to that seen in classical T cell mediated EAE. A humoral immune response to MBP was only detected in limited numbers of those rats with SAME.

Characterization of MBP–specific T cell lines from rats with same

As a consequence of these observations, the fine specificity of MBP-specific T cell lines from animals with SAME and EAE were analysed. For this purpose a panel of synthetic peptides from guinea pig MBP (Gp–MBP) representing the amino acid residues 69–84 that comprise the major encephalitogenic sequence for Lewis rats were used in proliferation assays (Liebert et al., 1990b). The MBP-specific T cell lines from both measles infected and MBP challenged rats revealed the same fine specificity and responded to *in vitro* stimulation with the encephalitogenic peptide S49 and S55 of Gp-MBP, but not to the non-encephalitogenic peptides S53, Leu4-S53 and 567 (Liebert et al., 1990b). This high degree of antigenic specificity is further supported by the failure of all these T cell lines to proliferate in the presence of MV particles, MV antigens or other control antigens or peptide sequences. In contrast, MV specific T cell lines only responded to MV proteins and not when MBP or synthetic peptides were added to the cultures.

Possible mechanisms of virus-induced autoimmune reactions

Studies in EAE have revealed that immunization of susceptible animals with MBP only leads to an autoimmune disease process of the CNS in conjunction with complete Freund's adjuvants. MBP immunization alone is ineffective which raises the question as to how MV may force the host to mount a strong cell-mediated immune response to brain antigen. Although the rat model has shown that immunization against MV leads to EAE there are certainly other ways by which the immune tolerance against host antigens can be overcome.

1. Target cell changes
   It has been proposed that during replication, the virus may incorporate host antigens into its envelope, insert, modify or expose cellular antigen on the cell surface. Such newly exposed antigens could be recognized as foreign by the host and could elicit a reaction in the same manner as any other previously unencountered protein (Hirsch and Proffitt, 1975). So far, definite proof of this hypothesis has not been presented although for certain virus infections this mechanism may induce autoimmune reactions (Notkins et al., 1984, Schattner and Rager-Zisman, 1990).

2. Interaction with lymphoid tissue
   Measles virus has a very strong tropism to lymphocytes and can infect T and B lymphocytes as well as macrophages. This interaction with the immune regulatory system *in vivo* could lead to the destruction of subpopulations of lymphocytes/monocytes or could, on the other hand, stimulate generations of lymphocyte clones that are autoreactive. In the rat model, the neurotropic MV does not seem to be lymphotropic since neither B or T lymphocytes of rats can be infected. However, it is well known that measles infection in man does alter host immune functions as well as antibody production

and that the disease is sometimes followed by serious complications such as exacerbations of tuberculosis (Cherry, 1981).

3. Molecular mimicry

   Molecular mimicry could be another mechanism by which an immune response is raised against certain viral antigens and which may in turn cross-react with normal host cell antigens (Oldstone and Notkins, 1986). Computer analysis of a variety of viral sequences revealed that several viruses including MV contain part of the human MBP sequence in their genome (Jahnke et al., 1985). Moreover, the immunization of rabbits with a synthetic peptide from such a sequence from hepatitis B virus polymerase led to the induction of EAE lesions in these animals (Fujinami and Oldstone, 1985). So far, MV specific T cell lines which recognize MBP have not been found in man or in animal experiments although one cannot exclude that this mechanism could play an important role in the pathogenesis of autoimmune reactions if similar structures of an infectious agent and a host cell protein share antigenic sites or interact with identical T cell receptors.

4. Does virus-mediated MHC class II induction trigger autoimmunity?

   Of particular interest for the development of an immunopathological reaction in the course of a CNS viral infection are the events of MHC class II induction on brain cells and a subsequent pathological response such as a delayed type sensitivity (DTH) reaction in genetically susceptible hosts. It has been established that major histocompatibility (MHC) antigens are expressed only at low levels or not at all on the majority of cells in the CNS (Hart and Fabre, 1981). There is evidence, however, that a number of glial cells may be induced to express MHC antigens by treatment with agents such as interferon γ *in vitro* (Wong et al., 1985) or as a result of an inflammatory reaction *in vivo*, presumably due to the release of interferon-γ by infiltrating T cells (Traugott et al., 1985). The problem, however, remains as to which factor(s) initiate(s) such a reaction in the CNS, since without the presence of MHC class II antigens, it is undoubtedly very difficult for CD4+ cells to recognize antigen, to become activated and to release lymphokines. Therefore, in a viral infection of the CNS, additional mechanisms probably operate to induce MHC antigen expression which would allow the T lymphocyte to find its target cell. With respect to MV, it has been shown that exposure of astrocytes in culture may lead to the expression of MHC class II antigen that can be further enhanced by the addition of tumor necrosis factor (Massa et al., 1986, 1987). Moreover, it has been found that astrocytes expressing class II antigen can present MBP to CD4[+] T lymphocytes (Fontana et al., 1984). Whether these events are important for the development of acute measles encephalitis in man or of SAME in the rat model is not known as well as the role of astrocytes and microglia in the presentation of autoantigens in virus-associated autoimmune diseases of the CNS.

Conclusions

The role of MV infections in the pathogenesis of several human diseases has elicited intense studies dealing with different aspects of MV associated disease processes. As summarized in this review, these include acute and late consequences of acute measles that are established in the presence or absence of the virus. Although progress has been made towards the pathogenesis of MV-induced autoimmune reactions and the regulation of MV gene expression in cells of neural origin, important questions concerning both conditions are far from being understood. Probably a main feature important for acute and late complications is the interaction of MV with peripheral blood mononuclear cells and, as a consequence, the MV associated interference with immune functions. The characteristic lymphopenia apparent during acute measles is characterized by a highly reduced population of CD4+ and CD8+ T cells. This depletion may be linked to virus-induced cytolysis as well as an infection-dependent inhibition of proliferation as observed in tissue culture experiments and in patients with acute measles. Yet, in spite of the pathogenetic role of the interaction of MV with peripheral blood mononuclear cells (PBMC) in MV associated diseases, little is known about the mechanism of MV induced immunosuppression and adequate experimental systems are not available. However, recently the human MV receptor complex has been identified and consists of at least two molecules, the membrane cofactor protein CD46 (Doerig et al., 1993, Naniche et al., 1993) and the cytoskeleton associated *m*embrane *o*rganizing *ex*ternal *s*pike prote*in* moesin (Dunster et al., 1994). Stable expression of CD46 already conferred susceptibility to several mouse cell lines including lymphocytic cells (Naniche et al., 1993). Infection with certain strains of MV has been associated with downregulation of CD46 from the surface of susceptible cell lines (Schneider-Schaulies et al., 1995), and that expression of the H protein was necessary and sufficient to exert this receptor modulation (Schneider-Schaulies et al., 1995, 1996). As the natural function of CD46 is to protect cells from complement mediated lysis, MV infected cells have been shown to reveal an enhanced sensitivity to activated complement (Schnorr et al., 1995). Although it is clear that sequences within the MV H protein are responsible for receptor modulation neither the mechanisms nor the association of this ability with MV virulence have been established yet.

As a major breakthrough to establish structure-function relationships for MV and host cell factors, a system allowing a reverse genetic approach for MV has been established (Radecke et al., 1995). Now it will be possible to assess MV gene functions by altering the viral genomic sequence. This approach will not only allow one to define specified viral gene functions, but also test directly for the ability of mutated MV genes, isolated from persistent human CNS infections to exert these functions, thus providing important insight into the pathogenesis of MV associated disease processes.

Acknowledgments

The authors are grateful to Deutsche Forschungsgemeinschaft, Bundesministerium für Forschung und Technologie and the Schweizerische Nationalfond for supporting the experimental work in their laboratories.

Bibliography

Andjaparidze, O. G., N. M. Chaplygina, N. N. Bogomolova, I. B. Koptyaeva, E. G. Nevryaeva, R. G. Filimova, and I. E. Tareeva (1989). Detection of measles virus genome in blood leucocytes of patients with certain autoimmune diseases. *Arch. Virol.* 105:287–291.

Antic, D., B. U. Lim, and C. Y. Kang (1992). Molecular characterization of the M genomic segment of the Seoul 80-39 virus: nucleotide and amino acid sequence comparisons with other hantaviruses reveal the evolutionary pathway. *Virus Res.* 19:47–58.

Baczko, K., J. Lampe, U. G. Liebert, U. Brinckmann, V. ter Meulen, J. Pardowitz, H. Budka, A. L. Cosby, S. Isserte, and B. K. Rima (1993). Clonal expansion of hypermutated measles virus in a SSPE brain. *Virology* 197:188–195.

Baczko, K., J. Pardowitz, B. K. Rima, and V. ter Meulen (1992). Constant and variable regions of measles virus proteins encoded by the nucleocapsid and phosphoprotein genes derived from lytic and persistent viruses. *Virology* 190:469–474.

Baczko, K., U. G. Liebert, M. A. Billeter, R. Cattaneo, H. Budka, and V. ter Meulen (1986). Expression of defective measles virus genes in brain tissues of patients with subacute sclerosing panencephalitis. *J. Virol.* 59:472–478.

Barrett, P., K. Koschel, M. Carter, and V. ter Meulen (1985). Effect of measles virus antibodies on a measles SSPE virus persistently infected C6 rat-glioma cell line. *J. Gen. Virol.* 66:1411–1421.

Basle, M. F., J. G. Fournier, S. Rozenblatt, A. Rebel, and M. Bouteille (1986). Measles virus RNA detected in Paget's disease bone tissue by *in situ* hybridization. *J. Gen. Virol.* 67:907–913.

Bass, B. L., and H. Weintraub (1987). A developmentally regulated activity that unwinds RNA duplexes. *Cell* 48:607–613.

Billeter, M. A. and R. Cattaneo (1991). Mutations and A/I hypermutations in: *"Measles virus persistent infections. The paramyxoviruses."* (D. Kingsbury, Ed.), pp. 323–345. Plenum, New York.

Billeter, M. A., R. Cattaneo, P. Spielhofer, K. Kaelin, M. Huber, A. Schmid, K. Baczko, and V. ter Meulen (1994). Generation and properties of measles virus mutations typically associated with subacute sclerosing panencephalitis. *Ann. NY Acad. Sci.* 724:367–377.

Cattaneo, R., and J. K. Rose (1993). Cell fusion by the envelope glycoproteins of persistent measles viruses which caused lethal human brain diseases. *J. Virol.* 67:1493–1502.

Cattaneo, R., A Schmid, P. Spielhofer, K. Kaelin, K. Baczko, V. ter Meulen, J. Pardowitz, S. Flanagan, B. K. Rima, S. A. Udem, and M. A. Billeter (1989). Mutated and hypermutated genes of persistent measles viruses which caused lethal human brain diseases. *Virology* 173:415–425.

Cattaneo, R., G. Rebmann, A. Schmid, K. Baczko, V. ter Meulen, and M. A. Billeter (1987a). Altered transcription of a defective measles virus genome derived from a diseased human brain. *EMBO J.* 6:681–687.

Cattaneo, R., G. Rebmann, K. Baczko, V. ter Meulen, and M. A. Billeter (1987b). Altered ratios of measles virus transcripts in diseased human brains. *Virology* 160:523–526.

Cherry, J. D. (1981). Measles, p. 1210–1230. *In* R. D. Feigin, and J. D. Cherry (ed.): *Textbook of Pediatric Infectious Diseases*, Vol. II Saunders, W. B., Philadelphia.

Cosby, S. L., S. Macquaid, M. J. Taylor, M. Bailey, B. K. Rima, S. J. Martin, and I. V. Allen (1989). Examination of eight cases of multiple sclerosis and 56 neurological and nonneurological controls for genomic sequences of measles virus. *J. Gen. Virol. 70*:2027–2036.

Cosby, S. L. (1993). Measles virus: A possible role in various diseases of unknown origin. *Microbiology Europe 5*:22–26.

Doerig, R. E., A Marcil, A. Chopra, and C. D. Richardson (1993). The human CD46 molecule is a receptor for measles virus (Edmonston strain). *Cell 75*:295–305.

Dunster, L. M., J. Schneider-Schaulies, S. Löffler, S. W. Lankes, R. Schwarz-Albiez, F. Lottspeich, and V. ter Meulen (1994). Moesin: A cell membrane protein linked with susceptibility to measles virus infection. *Virology 198*:265–274.

Ecker, A., V. ter Meulen, and S. Schneider-Schaulies (1995). Differentiation dependent regulation of unwinding/modifying activity for measles virus in neural cells. *J. Neurovirol. 1*:92–100.

Esolen, L. M., B. J. Ward, T. R. Moench, and D. E. Griffin (1993). Infection of monocytes during measles. *J. Inf. Dis. 168*:47–52.

Fontana, A., W. Fierz, and H. Wekerle (1984). Astrocytes present myelin basic protein to encephalitogenic T cell lines. *Nature 307*:273–276.

Fujinami, R. S., and M. B. A. Oldstone (1985). Amino acid homology and immune responses between the encephalitogenic site of myelin basic protein and virus: A mechanism for autoimmunity. *Science 230*:1043–1045.

Griffin, D. E., S. J. Cooper, R. L. Hirsch, R. T. Johnson, I. L. de Soriano, S. Roedenbeck, and A. Vaisberg (1985). Changes in plasma IgE levels during complicated and uncomplicated measles virus infections. *J. Allergy Clin. Immunol. 76*:206–213.

Griffin, D. E., B. J. Ward, E. Jauregui, R. T. Johnson, and A. Vaisberg (1989). Immune activation during measles. *N. Engl. J. Med. 320*:1667–1672.

Gustafson, T. L., A. W. Lievens, and P. A. Bourell (1987). Measles outbreak in a fully immunized secondary school population. *N. Engl. J. Med. 316*:717–724.

Haase, A. T., P. Ventura, C. G. Gibbs, and W. W. Tourtelotte (1981). Measles virus nucleotide sequences: detection by hybridization *in situ*. *Science 212*:672–675.

Hart, D. N. J., and J. W. Fabre (1981). Demonstration and characterization of Ia-positive dendritic cells in the interstitial tissues of rat heart and other tissues, but not brain. *J. Exp. Med. 154*:347–361.

Hirano, A. (1992). Subacute sclerosing panencephalitis virus dominantly interferes with replication of wild type measles virus in a mixed infection: implication for viral persistence. *J. Virol. 66*:1891–1898.

Hirano, A., M. Ayata, A. H. Wang and T. C. Wong (1993). Functional analysis of matrix proteins expressed from cloned genes of measles virus variants that cause subacute sclerosing panencephalitis reveals a common defect in nucleocapsid binding. *J. Virol. 67*:1848–1853.

Hirsch, M. S., and M. R. Proffitt (1975). Autoimmunity in viral infection, p. 419–434. *In* A. L. Notkins (ed.), *Viral Immunology and Immunopathology.* Academic Press, New York.

Itoyama, Y., and H. de F. Webster (1982). Immunocytochemical study of myelin-associated glycoprotein (MAG) and basic protein (BP) in acute experimental allergic encephalomyelitis (EAE). *J. Neuroimmunol. 3*:351–364.

Jahnke, U., E. H. Fischer, and E. C. Alvord (1985). Sequence homology between certain viral proteins and proteins related to encephalomyelitis and neuritis. *Science 229*:282–284.

Johnson, R. T., and D. E. Griffin (1986). Virus-induced autoimmune demyelinating disease of the CNS, p. 203–209. *In* A. L. Notkins, and M. B. A. Oldstone (ed.), *Concepts in Viral Pathogenesis II.* Springer Verlag, New York.

Johnson, R. T., D. E. Griffin, R. L. Hirsch, J. S. Wolinsky, S. Roedenbeck, S. I. L. Soriano, and A. Vaisberg (1984). Measles encephalomyelitis-clinical and immunologic studies. *N. Engl. J. Med. 310*:137–141.

Liebert, U. G., K. Baczko, H. Budka, and V. ter Meulen (1986). Restricted expression of measles virus proteins in brains from cases of subacute sclerosing panencephalitis. *J. Gen. Virol. 67*:2435–2444.

Liebert, U. G., and V. ter Meulen (1987). Virological aspects of measles virus induced encephalomyelitis in Lewis and BN rats. *J. Gen. Virol. 68*:1715–1722.

Liebert, U. G., C. Linington, and V. ter Meulen V. (1988). Induction of autoimmune reactions to myelin basic protein in measles virus encephalitis in Lewis rats. *J. Neuroimmunol. 17*:103–118.

Liebert, U. G., S. Schneider-Schaulies, K. Baczko and V. ter Meulen (1990a). Antibody-induced restriction of viral gene expression in measles encephalitis in rats. *J. Virol. 64*:706–713.

Liebert, U. G., G. A. Hashim, and V. ter Meulen (1990b). Characterization of measles virus-induced cellular autoimmune reactions against myelin basic protein in Lewis rats. *J. Neuroimmunol. 29*:139–147.

Massa, P. T., A. Schimpl, E. Wecker and V. ter Meulen (1987). Tumor necrosis factor amplifies measles virus-mediated Ia induction on astrocytes. *Proc. Natl. Acad. Sci. USA 84*:7242–7245.

Massa, P. T., R. Dörries, and V. ter Meulen (1986). Viral particles induce Ia antigen expression on astrocytes. *Nature 320*:543–546.

McKenna, M. J., and B. G. Mills (1989). Immunohistochemical evidence of measles virus antigens in active otosclerosis. *Otolaryngol. Head Neck Surg. 101*:415–421.

Moench, T. R., D. E. Griffin, C. R. Obriecht, A. Vaisberg and R. T. Johnson (1988). Distribution of measles virus antigen and RNA in acute measles with and without neurologic involvement. *J. Infect. Dis. 158*:433–442.

Murphy, D. G., Dimock, K., and C. Y. Kang (1991). Numerous transitions in human parainfluenza virus 3 RNA recovered from persistently infected cells. *Virology 181*:760–763.

Naniche, D., G. Varior-Krishnan, F. Cervoni, T. F. Wild, B. Rossi, C. Rabourdin-Combe, and D. Gerlier (1993). Human membrane cofactor protein (CD46) acts a cellular receptor for measles virus. *J. Virol.* 67:6025–6032.

Nishikura, K., C. Yoo, U. Kim, J. M. Murray, P. A. Estes, F. E. Cash and S. A. Liebhaber (1991). Substrate specificity of the dsRNA unwinding/modifying activity. *EMBO J.* 5:3523–3532.

Norrby, E., G. Enders-Ruckle, and V. ter Meulen (1975). Differences in the appearance of antibodies to structural components of measles virus after immunization with inactivated live virus. *J. Infect. Dis.* 262–269.

Notkins, A. L., T. Onodera, and B. S. Prabhaker (1984). Virus-induced autoimmunity, p. 210–215. *In* A. L. Notkins, and M. B. A. Oldstone (ed.), *Concepts in Viral Pathogenesis*. Springer Verlag, New York.

Ohuchi, M., R. Ohuchi, K. Mifune, T. Ishihara, and T. Ogawa (1987). Characterization of the measles virus isolated from the brain of a patient with immunosuppressive measles encephalitis. *J. Infect. Dis.* 156:436–441.

Oldstone, M. B. A., and A. L. Notkins (1986) Molecular mimicry, p. 195–202. *In* A. L. Notkins, and M. B. A. Oldstone (ed.), *Concepts in Viral Pathogenesis*. Springer Verlag, New York.

O'Hara, P. J., S. T. Nichol, F. M. Horodyski, and J. J. Holland (1984). Vesicular stomatitis virus defective interfering particles can contain extensive genomic sequence rearrangements and base substitutions. *Cell* 36:915–924.

Radecke F., P. Spielhofer, H. Schneider, K. Kälin, M. Huber, C. Dötsch, G. Christiansen, and M. A. Billeter (1995). Rescue of measles virus from cloned cDNA. *EMBO J.* 14:5773–5784.

Rager-Zisman, B., J. E. Egan, Y. Kress, and B. R. Bloom (1984). Isolation of cold-sensitive mutants of measles virus from persistently infected murine neuroblastoma cells. *J. Virol.* 51:845–855.

Raine, C. S. (1984). Biology of disease. Analysis of autoimmune demyelination: its impact upon Multiple Sclerosis. *Lab. Invest.* 50:608–635.

Rataul, S. M., A. Hirano, and T. C. Wong (1992). Irreversible modification of measles virus RNA *in vitro* by nuclear RNA-unwinding activity in human neuroblastoma cells. *J. Virol.* 66:1769–1773.

Rima, B. K. (1989). Comparison of amino acid sequences of the major structural proteins of the paramyxo- and morbilliviruses, p. 254–263. *In* B. W. J. Mahy and D. Kolakofsky (ed.) *Genetics and Pathogenicity of Negative Strand Viruses*. Elsevier, Amsterdam.

Robertson, D. A. F., E. C. Guy, S. L. Zhang, and R. Wright (1987). Persistent measles virus genome in autoimmune chronic active hepatitis. *Lancet ii*:9–11.

Roos, R. P., M. C. Graves, R.L. Wollman, R. R. Chilcote, and J. Nixon (1981). Immunologic and virologic studies of measles inclusion body encephalitis in an immunosuppressed host: the relationship to subacute sclerosing panencephalitis. *Neurology 31*:1263–1270.

Rota, J. S., K. B. Hummel, P. A. Rota, and W. J. Bellini (1992). Genetic variability of the glycoprotein genes of current wild type measles isolates. *Virology 188*:135–142.

Schattner, A., and B. Rager-Zisman (1990). Virus-induced autoimmunity. *Rev. Infect. Dis. 12*:204–222.

Schmid, A., P. Spielhofer, R. Cattaneo, K. Baczko, V. ter Meulen, and M. A. Billeter (1992). Subacute sclerosing panencephalitis is typically characterized by alterations in the fusion protein cytoplasmic domain of the persisting measles virus. *Virology 188*:910–915.

Schneider-Schaulies, S., U. G. Liebert, K. Baczko, R. Cattaneo, M. A. Billeter, and V. ter Meulen (1989). Restriction of measles virus gene expression in acute and subacute encephalitis of Lewis rats. *Virology 171*:525–534.

Schneider-Schaulies, S., U. G. Liebert, K. Baczko, and V. ter Meulen (1990). Restricted expression of measles virus in primary rat astroglial cells. *Virology 177*:802–806.

Schneider-Schaulies, S., and V. ter Meulen (1992). Molecular aspects of measles virus induced central nervous system diseases, p. 419–449. *In* R. P. Roos (ed.), *Molecular Neurovirology*. Humana Press Inc., Clifton, NJ.

Scheider-Schaulies, S., U. G. Liebert, Y. Segev, B. Rager-Zisman, M. Wolfson, and V. ter Meulen (1992). Antibody-dependent transcriptional regulation of measles virus in persistently infected neural cells. *J. Virol. 66*:5534–5541.

Schneider-Schaulies, S., J. Schneider-Schaulies, M. Bayer, S. Löffler, and V. ter Meulen (1993). Spontaneous and differentiation dependent regulation of measles virus gene expression in human glial cells. *J. Virol. 67*:3375–3383.

Schneider-Schaulies, S., A. Schuster, J. Schneider-Schaulies, M. Bayer, J. Pavlovic, and V. ter Meulen (1994). Cell type specific MxA-mediated inhibition of measles virus transcription in human brain cells. *J. Virol 68*: 6910–6917.

Schneider-Schaulies, J., J. J. Schnorr, U. Brinkmann, L. M. Dunster, K. Baczko, S. Schneider-Schaulies, and V. ter Meulen (1995). Receptor usage and differential downregulation of CD46 by measles virus wild type and vaccine strains. *Proc. Natl. Acad. Sci. 92*:3943–3947.

Schnorr, J. J., L. M. Dunster, R. Nanan, J. Schneider-Schaulies, S. Schneider-Schaulies, and V. ter Meulen (1995). Measles virus induced downregulation of CD46 is associated with enhanced sensitivity to complement mediated lysis of infected cells. *Europ. J. Immunol. 25*:976–984.

Schneider-Schaulies, J., J. J. Schnorr, J. Schlender, L. M. Dunster, S. Schneider-Schaulies, and V. ter Meulen (1996). Receptor (CD46) modulation and complement mediated lysis of uninfected cells after contact with measles virus-infected cells. *J. Virol. 70*:255–263.

Sheppard, R. D., C. S. Raine, M. B. Bornstein, and S. A. Udem (1986). Rapid degradation restricts measles virus matrix protein expression in a subacute sclerosing panencephalitis cell line. *Proc. Natl. Acad. Sci. USA 83*:7913–7917.

Sleat, D. E., N. F. Chikkala, S. Gautam, and A. K. Banerjee (1993). Restricted replication of vesicular stomatitis virus in T lymphocytes is coincident with a deficiency in a cellular protein kinase required for viral transcription. *J. Gen. Virol. 73*:3125–3132.

Taylor, M. J., E. Godfrey, K. Baczko, V. ter Meulen, T. F. Wild, and B. K. Rima (1991). Identification of several different lineages of measles virus. *J. Gen. Virol.* 72:83–88.

ter Meulen, V., and J. R. Stephenson (1983). The possible role of viral infections in MS and other related demyelinating diseases, p. 241–274. *In* J. F. Hallpike, C. W. M. Adams, and W. W. Tourtellotte (ed.) *Multiple Sclerosis.* Chapman & Hall, London.

ter Meulen, V., J. R. Stephenson, and H. W. Kreth (1983). Subacute sclerosing panencephalitis, p. 105–159. *In* H. Fraenkel-Conrat, and R. R. Wagner (ed.) *Comprehensive Virology.* Elsevier, Amsterdam.

Traugott, U., L. C. Scheinberg, and C. S. Raine (1985). On the presence of Ia-positive endothelial cells and astrocytes in multiple sclerosis lesions and its relevance to antigen presentation. *J. Neuroimmunol.* 8:1–14.

Vandenbark, A. A., T. Gill, and H. Offner (1985). A myelin basic protein-specific T cell line that mediates experimental allergic autoimmune encephalomyelitis. *J. Immunol.* 135:223–228.

Wagner, R. W., and K. Nishikura (1988). Cell cycle expression of RNA duplex unwindase activity in mammalian cells. *Mol. Cell. Biol.* 8:770–777.

Weinmann-Dorsch, C., and K. Koschel (1990). Coupling of viral membrane proteins to phosphatidylinositide signalling system. *FEBS Lett.* 247:185–188.

Wong, G. H. W., P. F. Bartlett, I. Clark-Lewis, J. L. McKimm-Breschkin, and J. W. Schrader (1985). Interferon-γ induces the expression of H-2 and Ia antigens on brain cells. *J. Neuroimmunol.* 7:255–278.

Wong, T. C., M. Ayata, S. Ueda, and A. Hirano (1991). Role of biased hypermutation in evolution of subacute sclerosing panencephalitis virus from progenitor acute measles virus. *J. Virol.* 65:2191–2199.

Yamamura, T., T. Namikawa, M. Endoh, T. Kunishita, and T. Tabira (1986). Experimental allergic encephaloyelitis induced by proteolipid apoprotein in Lewis rats. *J. Neuroimmunol.* 12:143–153.

Yoshikawa, Y., and K. Yamanouchi (1984). Effects of papaverine treatment of replication of measles virus in human neural and non-neural cells. *J. Virol.* 50:489–496.

6

Interactions of measles virus and the immune system

Diane E. Griffin, Brian J. Ward, and Lisa M. Esolen
Johns Hopkins University
School of Medicine
Baltimore, MD 21205, USA

In the normal host measles virus causes an acute, self-limited infection and lifelong immunity to reinfection. In order to understand how and why measles virus occasionally becomes persistent it is useful to determine the nature of the immune response associated with successful clearance of virus as a basis for a better understanding of measles and comparison with the immune response during persistent infection.

The rash and the appearance of the immune response

One of the hallmarks of acute measles is the characteristic maculopapular erythematous rash. Histologically, the rash is composed of infected epidermal, dermal and capillary endothelial cells and of infiltrating mononuclear cells (Suringa et al. 1970; Olding-Stenkvist and Bjorvatn, 1976; Kimura et al. 1975). The infiltrating lymphocytes and monocytes are responding to virus infection in an immunologically specific fashion and this inflammatory response is a direct manifestation of the cellular immune response to measles virus-infected cells. The onset of the rash is also coincident with the appearance of antibody to various viral proteins (Graves et al., 1984; Bech, 1959) (Fig. 1). The earliest and most abundant antibody is to the N protein, but antibodies to H and F appear soon there-

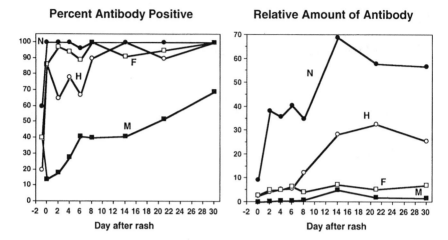

Figure 1 Frequency and amount of antibody to individual measles virus proteins relative to the onset of the rash. Adapted with permission from Graves et al., 1984.

after. Antibodies to H and N increase substantially during the second week. Although essentially all patients develop antibody to F after the first week, the amounts of antibody are lower than to either H or N. The M protein appears to be less immunogenic since a substantial number of individuals do not develop detectable antibody and the amounts of antibody are low (Graves et al. 1984).

Virus clearance

The rash lasts 3–5 days and virus clearance occurs during this time. Virus can be detected both in peripheral blood mononuclear cells and in various tissues early during the eruption, but is not detectable by routine techniques such as virus isolation, immunohistochemical staining and *in situ* hybridization one week later (Ruckle and Rogers, 1957; Forthal et al. 1992; Gresser and Chany, 1963). Even in tissues acquired at autopsy from individuals dying of measles, virus cannot be detected if death occurred after the rash had faded (Moench et al. 1988). Therefore, in most children dying of measles there is little evidence that death is due to uncontrolled replication of measles virus. Rare individuals with compromised immune function may not develop a rash and have persistent infection that progresses to giant cell pneumonia or inclusion body encephalitis due to failure to clear virus (Enders et al. 1959).

Complications and immunologic abnormalities

Most of the mortality, as well as the morbidity, during measles is due to a variety of complications that occur in otherwise immunocompetent individuals. Early textbooks of medicine described reactivation of tuberculosis and diarrhea, otitis media and pneumonia caused by secondary bacterial and viral infections are common complications of measles (Beckford et al. 1985; Miller, 1964; Greenberg et al. 1991). Therefore, reactivation of previous infections and increased susceptibility to new infections are characteristic features of measles and are thought to be due to the immunosuppression that occurs during this disease.

An additional important complication of measles is postinfectious or acute disseminated encephalomyelitis, a demyelinating disease most likely to be autoimmune in etiology (Miller, 1964; Johnson et al. 1984; Litvak et al. 1943). Both infectious and autoimmune complications occur during the rash or during the first few weeks after resolution of the rash.

During this same period of time multiple immunologic abnormalities can be objectively identified. The loss of skin test responses to tuberculin was first described around the turn of the century by von Pirquet (von Pirquet, 1908). This has been subsequently confirmed in a number of studies (Tamashiro et al. 1987). Another well-recognized laboratory indication of decreased immune responsiveness during measles is the diminution in proliferation of cultured lymphocytes in response to mitogens such as phytohemagglutinin (Hirsch et al. 1984). Both of these abnormalities often persist for weeks after apparent recovery from measles.

Therefore, a paradoxical situation exists in measles. The cellular and humoral antiviral immune response is effective in clearing virus from blood and tissues and in establishing lifelong immunity to reinfection. This appropriate response to a systemic viral infection is superimposed on a wide variety of immunologic abnormalities that lead to increased susceptibility to other infections, autoimmune disease, loss of delayed

type hypersensitivity skin test responses and depressed *in vitro* lymphoproliferative responses.

To investigate how measles may be affecting the immune response we
have addressed three related questions: (1) what cells relevant to the immune response are infected by measles virus, (2) what cells are immunologically activated and (3) what cytokines are activated cells producing?

Infection of mononuclear cells

As assessed from autopsy studies by immunohistochemical staining and
in situ hybridization, the types of cells infected by measles virus include
epithelial cells, endothelial cells and histiocytes (Moench et al. 1988). Virus can be cultured from peripheral blood leukocytes (Papp, 1937; Forthal et al. 1992). In culture, T cell, B cell and monocytic cell lines all
support measles virus replication (Joseph et al. 1975; Sullivan et al.
1975). Analysis of fractionated leukocytes from patients with acute
measles for measles virus RNA using the reverse transcriptase-polymerase chain reaction has identified the monocyte as the primary leukocyte
infected *in vivo* (Fig. 2) (Esolen et al. 1993). This fact was confirmed by
double staining of the cells. Therefore, although T lymphocyte function is
clearly affected during measles, there is little evidence that this is due to
virus infection of these cells *per se*.

The data do suggest, however, that monocyte function may be directly
affected by infection. During *in vitro* culture of peripheral blood mononuclear cells (PBMC) from patients with measles, IL-1β is produced in normal amounts while TNFα production is decreased (Ward et al. 1991).
This abnormality can be reproduced by infecting monocyte cell lines *in
vitro* with measles virus and measuring the cytokines produced in response to lipopolysaccharide (Leopardi et al. 1992). TNFα is a proin-
flammatory cytokine and inadequate production of this cytokine could
lead to abnormalities of *in vitro* proliferation of PBMC and *in vivo* recruitment of mononuclear cells into areas of inflammation. Expression of
MHC class II antigens is increased, but the ability of infected monocytes
to present antigens other than measles antigens to T cells is impaired
(Leopardi et al. 1993). Therefore, some of the immunologic abnormalities in measles may be related directly to measles virus infection of mono-

Adherent cells

Nonadherent cells

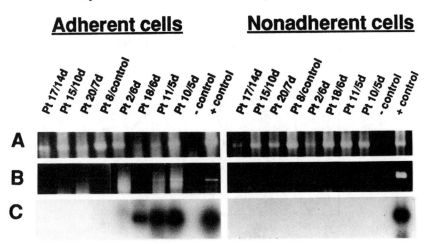

Figure 2 Analysis of measles virus infection of peripheral blood mononuclear cells by reverse transcriptase-polymerase chain reaction showing that virus can be detected only in adherent cells. Reproduced, with permission, from Esolen et al. 1993.

cytes. However, explaining T cell abnormalities may be somewhat more complicated.

T cell function during measles

To determine how T cells are functioning during measles we first determined what cells were activated at various times during infection. During the period of the rash spontaneous proliferation of PBMC occurs, suggesting *in vivo* activation of the cells (Arneborn and Biberfeld, 1983) (Fig. 3). Analysis of the types of cells proliferating shows that B cells, CD4 and CD8 T cells and monocytes are all activated (Ward et al. 1990). The relative proportions of each of these populations remain essentially unchanged so shifts in ratios of CD4 and CD8 T cells do not explain the immunologic abnormalities seen (Arneborn and Biberfeld, 1983; Griffin et al. 1986; Ward et al. 1990).

To examine the function of the different T cell populations in more detail several types of analyses have been performed. Activation of CD8 T

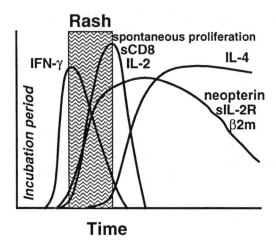

Figure 3 Schematic diagram of the changes in immunologic parameters occurring in the blood during natural measles in relation to appearance of the rash.
Reproduced with permission from Griffin et al., 1994.

cells has been demonstrated by isolation of measles virus-specific CD8
cytotoxic T cells from blood (Kreth et al. 1979; Sissons et al. 1985; van
Binnendijk et al. 1990) and demonstration of elevated levels of soluble
CD8 in plasma during the rash (Griffin et al. 1989). This is consistent
with the hypothesis that CD8+ T cells are important for clearing virus
from tissues by lysing virus-infected cells expressing MHC class I antigens. Correlation of the soluble CD8 levels in plasma and the detection of
virus in PBMCs suggests that once virus is cleared activation of CD8+ T
cells decreases (Griffin et al. 1989; Esolen et al. 1993).

Activation of CD4+ T cells has been demonstrated by finding CD4+ T
cells that proliferate in response to inactivated measles virus and by demonstration of elevated levels of soluble CD4 in the plasma of individuals
with measles (van Binnendijk et al. 1989; van Binnendijk et al. 1990).
The time course of CD4+ T cell activation indicates that it is initiated at a
similar time, but is more prolonged than that for CD8+ T cells, lasting
well beyond the disappearance of the rash and apparent clearance of virus
(Griffin and Ward, 1993) (Fig. 3).

After initial antigen stimulation, CD4+ T cells produce a broad array of cytokines including large amounts of IL-2. As T cells are restimulated with antigen and become fully differentiated they tend to narrow the range of cytokines produced and consequently narrow their functional capacities. Type 1 CD4+ T cells produce IL-2, IFN-γ and lymphotoxin (TNFβ). These cells are primarily involved in classic cellular immune responses and delayed type hypersensitivity skin test responses (Mosmann and Coffman, 1987). The lymphokines produced are important for macrophage activation (IFN-γ), lymphocyte proliferation (IL-2) and cellular cytotoxicity (TNFβ).

In contrast, type 2 CD4+ T cells produce IL-4, IL-5 and IL-10. These cytokines are important for B cell proliferation and differentiation leading to antibody production. Therefore, these cells are the primary providers of B cell help. In addition, IL-4 and IL-10 act to downregulate macrophage function and block the effects of IFN-γ (Mosmann and Coffman, 1987).

During measles the activation of T cells and production of cytokines is sufficient to allow these secreted products, as well as many solubilized cell surface molecules to be measured in plasma (Fig. 3). During the time of the rash IL-2 and IFN-γ are both elevated, but decline rapidly (Griffin and Ward, 1993; Griffin et al. 1990). These cytokines are postulated to be products of Th0 (IL-2) and CD8 (IFN-γ) T cells. Soluble IL-2 receptor, β2microglobulin and neopterin all become increased during the rash and decline slowly over the next few weeks (Griffin et al. 1992; Griffin et al. 1990; Griffin et al. 1989). Neopterin is a product of IFN-γ-activated macrophages, and macrophages are a likely source of the β2microglobulin as well. Soluble IL-2 receptor is a product of IL-2-activated T cells. The more prolonged time course of elevation of the levels of these products of activated macrophages and T cells in plasma suggests that even though IL-2 and IFN-γ have returned to normal (undetectable) levels in plasma, these cytokines continue to be produced and act locally in tissue well after the rash has resolved.

The time course for increase in plasma levels of IL-4 is of a third pattern. There is no evidence of IL-4 increase during the rash, but levels rise in many individuals within a few days and this increase continues for several weeks (Griffin and Ward, 1993). IL-4 is produced by type 2 CD4 T

In vitro production of IL-4

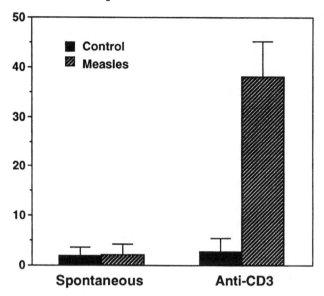

Figure 4 Production of IL-4 in response to stimulation with antibody to CD3 by peripheral blood mononuclear cells from patients recovering from measles. Adapted, with permission, from Griffin et al., 1993.

cells and elevated plasma levels suggest prolonged activation of this T cell subtype. Since IL-4 suppresses the activity of type 1 CD4 cells it is postulated that preferential activation of type 2 CD4 T cells may contribute to the depression of delayed type hypersensitivity skin test responses and other parameters of cellular immunity, at the same time that B cell production of antibody is being encouraged.

To determine whether IL-4 contributes to decreased lymphoproliferation in response to phytohemagglutinin during measles, levels of IL-4 were measured in supernatant fluids of PBMC cultured from individuals recovering from measles (Fig. 4). IL-4 was increased compared to supernatant fluids from control cells, and addition of antibody to IL-4 improved proliferative responses in individuals studied after clearance of the rash (Griffin and Ward, 1993). These data suggest that type 2 CD4 T cells and IL-4 specifically contribute to the immunosuppression seen after measles.

This pattern of T cell response is consistent with other observations of immunologic memory in measles. One of the most characteristic features of longterm measles immunity is a persistent, high level of measles virus-specific antibody. Features of the measles virus-specific T cell response include limited *in vitro* proliferation of PBMC and lack of positive skin test responses to measles virus antigens (Fulginiti and Arthur, 1969; Nelson et al. 1966; McFarland and McFarlin, 1979). We propose that the measles virus-specific CD4 T cell response is predominantly type 2 leading to excellent antibody responses, poor classic cellular immune responses and global suppression of macrophage and type 1 CD4 T cell responses for a prolonged period of time after measles. It will be of interest to compare this pattern of measles virus-specific immunity during acute infection to that which exists during persistent infection.

References

Arneborn, P. and Biberfeld, G. (1983). T lymphocyte subpopulations in relation to immunosuppression in measles and varicella. *Infect. Immun. 39*, 29–37.

Bech, V. (1959). Studies on the development of complement fixing antibodies in measles patients. *J. Immunol. 83*, 267–275.

Beckford, A. P., Kaschula, R. O. C., and Stephen, C. (1985). Factors associated with fatal cases of measles: A retrospective autopsy study. *S. Afr. Med. J. 68*, 858–863.

Enders, J. F., McCarthy, K., Mitus, A., and Cheatham, W. J. (1959). Isolation of measles virus at autopsy in cases of giant cell pneumonia without rash. *N. Eng. J. Med. 261*, 875–881.

Esolen, L. M., Ward, B. J., Moench, T. R., and Griffin, D. E. (1993). Infection of monocytes during measles. *J. Infect. Dis. 168*, 47–52.

Forthal, D. N., Aaranes, S., Blanding, J., and Maza, L. (1992). Degree and length of viremia in adults with measles. *J. Infect. Dis. 166*, 421–424.

Fulginiti, V. A. and Arthur, J. H. (1969). Altered reactivity to measles virus. *J. Pediatr. 75*, 609–616.

Graves, M., Griffin, D. E., Johnson, R. T., Hirsch, R. L., Lindo de Soriano, I., Roedenbeck, S., and Vaisberg, A. (1984). Development of antibody to measles virus polypeptides during complicated and uncomplicated measles virus infections. *J. Virol. 49*, 409–412.

Greenberg, B. L., Sack, R. B., Salazar-Lindo, E., Budge, E., Gutierrez, M., Campos, M., Vaisberg, A., Leon-Barua, R., Yi, A., Maurutia, D., Gomez, M., Lindo, I., and Jauregui, E. (1991). Measles-associated diarrhea in hospitalized children in Lima, Peru: Pathogenic agents and impact on growth. *J. Infect. Dis. 163*, 495–502.

Gresser, I. and Chany, C. (1963). Isolation of measles virus from the washed leucocytic fraction of blood. *Proc. Soc. Exp. Biol. Med. 113*, 695–698.

Griffin, D. E., Moench, T. R., Johnson, R. T., Lindo de Soriano, I., and Vaisberg, A. (1986). Peripheral blood mononuclear cells during natural measles virus infection: Cell surface phenotypes and evidence for activation. *Clin. Immunol. Immunopathol. 40*, 305–312.

Griffin, D. E., Ward, B. J., and Esolen, L. M. (1994). Pathogenesis of measles virus infection: An hypothesis for altered immune responses. *J. Infect. Dis. 170*, Suppl. 1, 524–31.

Griffin, D. E., Ward, B. J., Jauregui, E., Johnson, R. T., and Vaisberg, A. (1989). Immune activation during measles. *N. Eng. J. Med. 320*, 1667–1672.

Griffin, D. E., Ward, B. J., Jauregui, E., Johnson, R. J., and Vaisberg, A. (1990). Immune activation during measles: interferon-gamma and neopterin in plasma and cerebrospinal fluid in complicated and uncomplicated disease. *J. Infect. Dis. 161*, 449–453.

Griffin, D. E., Ward, B. J., Jauregui, E., Johnson, R. T., and Vaisberg, A. (1992). Immune activation during measles: Beta-2-microglobulin in plasma and cerebrospinal fluid in complicated and uncomplicated disease. *J. Infect. Dis. 166*, 1170–1173.

Griffin, D. E. and Ward, B. J. (1993). Differential CD4 T cell activation in measles. *J. Infect. Dis. 168*, 275–281.

Hirsch, R. L. Griffin, D. E., Johnson, R. T., Cooper, S. J., Lindo de Soriano, I., Roedenbeck, S., and Vaisberg, A. (1984). Cellular immune responses during complicated and uncomplicated measles virus infections of man. *Clin. Immunol. Immunopathol. 31*, 1–12.

Johnson, R. T., Griffin, D. E., Hirsch, R. L., Wolinsky, J. S., Roedenbeck, S., Lindo de Soriano, I., and Vaisberg, A. (1984). Measles encephalomyelitis—clinical and immunologic studies. *N. Eng. J. Med. 310*, 137–141.

Joseph, B. S., Lamperts, P. W., and Oldstone, M. B. A. (1975). Replication and persistence of measles virus in defined subpopulations of human leukocytes. *J. Virol. 16*, 1638–1649.

Kimura, A., Tosaka, K., and Nakao, T. (1975). Measles rash. I. Light and electron microscopic study of skin eruptions. *Arch. Virol. 47*, 295–307.

Kreth, H. W., ter Meulen, V., and Eckert, G. (1979). Demonstration of HLA restricted killer cells in patients with acute measles. *Med. Microbiol. Immunol. 165*, 203–214.

Leopardi, R., Vainionpää, R., Hurme, M., Siljander, P., and Salmi, A. A. (1992). Measles virus infection enhances Il-1β but reduces tumor necrosis factor-α expression in human monocytes. *J. Immunol. 149*, 2397–2401.

Leopardi, R., Ilonen, J., Mattila, L., and Salmi, A. A. (1993). Effect of measles virus infection on MHC class II expression and antigen presentation in human monocytes. *Cell. Immunol. 147*, 388–396.

Litvak, A. M., Sands, I. J., Gibel, H. (1943). Encephalitis complicating measles: Report of fifty-six cases with followup studies in thirty-two. *Amer. J. Dis. Child. 65,* 265–295.

McFarland, H. F. and McFarlin, D. E. (1979). Cellular immune response to measles, mumps, and vaccinia viruses in multiple sclerosis. *Ann. Neurol. 6,* 101–106.

Miller, D. L. (1964). Frequency of complications of measles, 1963. *Brit. Med. J. 2,* 75–78.

Moench, T. R., Griffin, D. E., Obriecht, C. R., Vaisberg, A. J., and Johnson, R. T. (1988). Acute measles in patients with and without neurological involvement: Distribution of measles virus antigen and RNA. *J. Infect. Dis. 158,* 433–442.

Mosmann, T. R. and Coffman, R. L. (1987). Two types of mouse helper T cell clone: Implications for immune regulation. *Immunol. Today 8,* 223–227.

Nelson, J. D., Sandusky, G., and Peck, F. B. (1966). Measles skin test and serologic response to intradermal measles antigen. *J. Amer. Med. Assoc. 198,* 185–186.

Olding-Stenkvist, E. and Bjorvatn, B. (1976). Rapid detection of measles virus in skin rashes by immunofluorescence. *J. Infect. Dis. 134,* 463–469.

Papp, K. (1937). Fixation der virus morbilleux aux leucocytes du sand des la periode d'incubation de la maladie. *Bull. Acad. Med. Paris 117,* 46–51.

Ruckle, G. and Rogers, K. D. (1957). Studies with measles virus. II. Isolation of virus and immunologic studies in persons who have had the natural disease. *J. Immunol. 78,* 341–355.

Sissons, J. G. P., Colby, S. D., Harrison, W. O., and Oldstone, M. B. A. (1985). Cytotoxic lymphocytes generated *in vivo* with acute measles virus infection. *Clin. Immunol. Immunopathol. 34,* 60–68.

Sullivan, J. L., Barry, D. W., Lucas, S. J., and Albrecht, P. (1975). Measles infection of human mononuclear cells. I. Acute infection of peripheral blood lymphocytes and monocytes. *J. Exp. Med. 142,* 773–784.

Suringa, D. W. R., Bank, L. J., and Ackerman, B. (1970). Role of measles virus in skin lesions and Koplik's spots. *N. Engl. J. Med. 283,* 1139–1142.

Tamashiro, V. G., Perez, H. H., and Griffin, D. E. (1987). Prospective study of the magnitude and duration of changes in tuberculin reactivity during complicated and uncomplicated measles. *Pediat. Infect. Dis. J. 6,* 451–454.

van Binnendijk, R., Poelen, M. C. M., deVries, P., Voorma, H. O., Osterhaus, A. D. M. E., and Uytdehaag, F. G. C. M. (1989). Measles virus-specific human T cell clones. Characterization of specificity and function of CD4 helper/cytotoxic and CD8+ cytotoxic T cell clones. *J. Immunol. 142,* 2847–2854.

van Binnendijk, R. S., Poelen, M. C. M., Kuijpers, K. C., Osterhaus, A. D. M. E., and Uytdehaag, F. G. C. M. (1990). The predominance of CD8+ T cells after infection with measles virus suggests a role for CD8+ class I MHC-restricted cytotoxic T lymphocytes (CTL) in recovery from measles. *J. Immunol. 144,* 2394–2399.

von Pirquet, C. (1908). Verhalten der kutanen tuberkulin-reaktion wahrend der Masern. *Deutsch. Med. Wochenschr. 34,* 1297–1300.

Ward, B. J., Johnson, R. T., Vaisberg, A., Jaurequi, E., and Griffin, D. E. (1990). Spontaneous proliferation of peripheral mononuclear cells in natural measles virus infection: Identification of dividing cells and correlation with mitogen responsiveness. *Clin. Immunol. Immunopathol.* 55, 315–326.

Ward, B. J., Johnson, R. T., Vaisberg, A. Jauregui, E., and Griffin, D. E. (1991). Cytokine production *in vitro* and the lymphoproliferative defect of natural measles virus infection. *Clin. Immunol. Immunopathol.* 61, 236–248.

7

Persistence of measles in a vaccinated population

William J. Bellini, Ph.D.
Department of Health and Human Services
Public Health Service
Centers for Disease Control and Prevention
Division of Viral and Rickettsial Diseases
Atlanta, GA 30333, USA

The resurgence of measles disease in the United States from 1989 to 1991 took the public health community by surprise. Despite major vaccination campaigns in the late 1970s and early 1980s to eliminate measles from the United States, greater than 60,000 reported cases and 150 measles-associated deaths occurred over this three-year period. The reasons surrounding the resurgence of measles in the U.S. population, although not completely understood, can arguably be considered to be the same as those involved in persistence of measles in a vaccinated population.

The epidemiological data presented in Figure 1 is a composite of the number of reported cases of measles between 1980 and 1994 and a summary of the age distribution and vaccination status of reported measles cases during the first 26 weeks of 1989 (Figure 1, inset; CDC, 1989). In 1980, there were about 14,000 cases of measles reported in the United States. This compares with the 500,000 to 600,000 cases that were routinely observed in the prevaccine era. With the introduction of vaccine in 1963, and finally with the use of the Attenuvax vaccine (the only licensed vaccine in the United States) beginning in 1972, the number of cases dropped precipitously. Until recently, the lowest number of cases reported

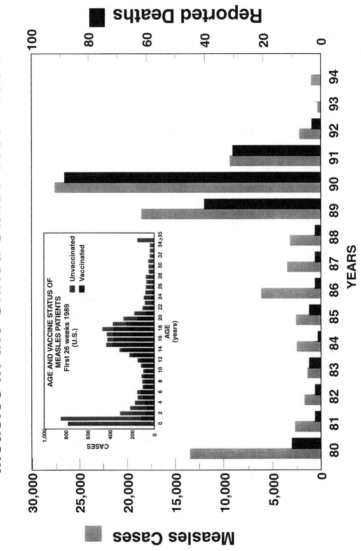

Figure 1   Reported measles cases and associated deaths in the United States from 1980 to 1994. Inset: Distribution of measles cases reported in the first 26 weeks of 1989 with respect to age and vaccine status.

was 1400 in 1983, but there was never a sustained number of reporting periods in that year with no measles cases reported. Only 500 of these cases could be traced to imported cases, whereas the remainders were assumed to be endemic. Most of the cases occurred in school- and college-aged individuals with little spread into the population under five years of age. From 1983 to 1988, the number of cases slowly increased. Then, between 1989 and 1990 a cumulative 55,000 cases of measles were reported. Over the 1989 to 1991 resurgent period more than 60,000 cases and 150 measles-associated deaths were accumulated, coupled with the highest complication and hospitalization rate and the highest fatality/case ratio ever reported for measles (Atkinson et al., 1992).

For the first twenty-six weeks period of 1989 (Figure 1, inset) about 40% of all cases occurred in persons 12 to 21 years-of-age that should, in fact, have been vaccinated. This finding was usual, for this same age group appeared to be involved in smaller outbreaks since 1980. Both primary and secondary vaccine failure (waning immunity) were cited as reasons for the measles observed in this population (Edmonson et al., 1990). Of greater concern was the finding that children aged less than 15 months could account for as much as 20 percent of the total cases. Those cases could not have been prevented by vaccination, since the Measles-Mumps-Rubella (MMR) vaccination is recommended only after 12 to 15 months-of-age. The age at which measles vaccine is administered stems from studies which have shown that maternal antibody is long lived in infants and the antibody appears to interfere with immunization up until that age (Albrecht et al., 1977). It was assumed, however, that the individual would also be protected from disease during this same time period.

A detailed look at the first twenty-six weeks of the resurgent period helped define some of the possible reasons for the renewed measles activity. First was the possibility that overall vaccine coverage was lower than anticipated, although surveillance measures indicated that vaccine coverage in most settings was in excess of 80%. Second was the possibility that the frequency of primary vaccine failure was somehow increasing, implying a problem with vaccine stability and/or potency. Third was the suggestion that secondary vaccine failure might be responsible for the accumulation of measles susceptible individuals in the 12 to 20 age group. Finally, based on marked increases in morbidity and mortality of reported measles cases during the resurgent period, genetic changes resulting in more virulent strains of measles virus were also considered.

Failure to vaccinate

It was surprising to learn that most of the large outbreaks in the inner cities arose because vaccine coverage had dropped to below 60%. Large preschool outbreaks occurring in Houston, Chicago, Los Angeles, New York City and Dallas were found to involve unvaccinated black and Hispanic children, usually under the age of two (CDC, 1991).

Another factor found to affect measles infection in children less than 15 months-of-age was whether or not their mothers were vaccinated or had natural measles. The mothers of many infants who developed measles infections less than one year-of-age were born after 1957, and thus were more likely to have been vaccinated. Indeed we and others found that children born of vaccinated mothers had less maternal antibody to measles and were seronegative for measles antibody by seven months-of-age (Pabst et al., 1992, Bromberg et al., 1994). Although this increased window of susceptibility certainly exists, further work is necessary to determine whether vaccine efficacy is as good at 7 months as compared with 12–15 months.

Primary vaccine failure

Historically, measles vaccine efficacy has been determined to be in excess of 95%. Of course this might vary a bit depending upon the nature of the assay used to make the determination of seroconversion. Using a recently developed sensitive IgM capture EIA (Hummel et al., 1992), vaccine efficacy was measured in 2000 children receiving MMR for the first time at 12 to 15 months-of-age. Only 2.0% of these children failed to seroconvert after vaccination. Interestingly, the vast majority of these children (all but 2) seroconverted when again given vaccine. The widely accepted view is that seroconversion correlates favorably with protection, but we also know that failure to seroconvert does not always indicate that an individual is necessarily susceptible to measles infection. Regardless, primary vaccine failure probably was not a major factor in either the resurgence or the persistence of measles in the population.

Secondary vaccine failure

The occurrence of clinically defined measles in persons, years after receiving live virus vaccine, has been attributed to primary vaccine failure due to insufficient primary antigenic stimulation, as well as secondary vaccine failure due to a putative loss of protective antibody or waning immunity. In clinical measles cases with a history of vaccination, the appearance of a primary IgM antibody response followed by an IgG response would be an indication of primary vaccine failure or failure to immunize. However, a secondary or anamnestic response, i.e., a rapid and heightened IgG response without detectable IgM has been taken as an indication of secondary vaccine failure or waning immunity.

Reports of measles outbreaks that have described cases of primary and secondary vaccine failure have often been based solely on the detection of specific IgM antibodies (Edmonson et al., 1990). Depending on the sensitivity and specificity of the assay employed, and the timing of specimen collection, measles cases could be misclassified, leading to a misinterpretation of the underlying cause of vaccine failure. In a recent study from this laboratory, the aforementioned sensitive measles IgM capture enzyme immunoassay (EIA) was used to evaluate the suitability of IgM as an indicator of primary and secondary antibody responses in persons receiving primary and secondary measles vaccination and in persons with natural measles virus infection (Erdman et al., 1993).

Of 32 nonimmune children receiving primary measles vaccination, 31(97%) developed IgM antibodies consistent with a primary antibody response. Of 21 previously vaccinated children with low levels of preexisting IgG antibodies who responded to revaccination, none developed detectable IgM antibodies, whereas 33 of 35 (94%) with no detectable preexisting IgG antibodies developed an IgM response. In this same study, of a sample of 57 measles cases with a prior history of vaccination, 55 (96%) had detectable IgM antibodies. Of these, 30 (55%) were classified as having a primary antibody response and 25 (45%) a secondary antibody response based on differences in their ratios of IgM to IgG antibodies. An IgM to IgG ratio greater than one correlated with more severe clinical symptoms (the majority met the established clinical case definition). An IgM to IgG ratio less than one correlated with less severe symptoms. These findings suggest that 1) an IgM response follows primary measles vaccination in the immunologically naive, 2) an IgM response is absent on revaccination of those previously immunized, and 3) an IgM response may follow clinical measles virus infection independent of prior immunization status. There is also evidence to suggest that close case contacts who have a history of natural infection, and have a resident IgG response, may also develop an IgM response to currently circulating virus (Mellinger et al., unpublished observation).

The major question remains whether or not these sub-clinical or inapparent infections are transmissible. If this can be proven to be the case, then we will have identified a mechanism by which measles virus can persist in a vaccinated population as an inapparent infection and then be transmitted to susceptible individuals by spreading the infection from a sub-clinically ill individual. Further investigation is necessary to provide a clear answer to this very important question.

Genetic variability of measles virus

As stated earlier, the possibility that genetic variants of measles virus were somehow involved in the resurgence appeared important to investigate because of the increase in the case fatality ratio, increased rate of hospitalization and the large number of measles cases that resulted in complications. Taken together these observations suggested increased virulence of the circulating measles virus, and suggested that changes in virulence might be reflected in the nucleotide sequences of the N, H and F genes of the wild viruses when compared with comparable regions of vaccine strains.

We first determined the degree of genetic heterogeneity among nine vaccine strains of measles virus. Most of these strains had the Edmonston strain (Enders et al., 1957) as their progenitor virus. Nucleotide sequence analysis of these strains supported the view that regardless of the passage history, the AIK-C, Schwarz, Moraten, Leningrad 16, Zagreb, and a strain we referred to as wild Edmonston (kindly provided by Paul Albrecht) were all very closely related. In fact even the most divergent strains, CAM-70 and Shanghai-191, were only 12 and nine nucleotides different from the wild Edmonston strain, respectively. The nucleoprotein gene sequence analysis resulted in similar conclusions. Given that most of the vaccine strains were isolated from nature in the fifties and early sixties, these results suggested that either there existed a single genotype of measles during that era, or that this genotype represented a dominant one or one that is easily isolated in cell culture. Measles virus was quite similar in the 1950s and 1960s, the time period over which most of the parent strains were isolated (Rota et al., 1994a).

In contrast, the genetic relationships determined from the sequence information of the H genes of wild measles viruses isolated in 1977, 1983 through 1989 implied a progressive evolution in wild-type measles viruses. There appeared to be a temporally related accumulation of nucleotide and amino acid changes in the H genes of the wildtype viruses. For each of the 1988–89 wildtype viruses, approximately 35% of the H base changes resulted in predicted amino acid substitutions (Rota et al., 1994b). The majority of these amino acid changes were situated in close proximity to the region spanning amino acid residues 167–241, where the five potential glycosylation sites are located. A potential new glycosylation site was identified near the carboxyl-terminus of the H at amino acid position 416 (Figure 2). Initially it was believed that the use of this site might account for the larger apparent size of the H protein of the wild viruses from 1983 through 1989 relative to vaccine or the 1977 viruses. However, endo-F treatment resulted in the same size differential of the unglycosylated forms of the protein, indicating that the size difference was due to the amino acid composition rather than glycosylation. Interestingly, Sakata and coworkers have identified three types of measles viruses containing H proteins of different electrophoretic mobilities in a collection of wild–type isolates. The small (S) type H variant dominated in Japan during 1983–1984 outbreaks, but was replaced by the medium (M) and large (L) variants between 1984 and 1990. They also found the nucleotide change that predicted a new potential glycosylation site at position 416 associated with the M and L variants (Sakata et al., 1993).

The nonrandom distribution of the conserved coding changes observed in the H coding sequence of all three of the 1988–89 wild-type viruses as well as the 1983 isolate may be indicative of selective pressure for these changes. Moreover, the paucity of third position changes also implied that some sort of selection was exerted. The identification of the protein,

Hemagglutinin Amino Acid Changes Predicted
From 1989-1991 U.S. Wildtype Measles Virus Sequences

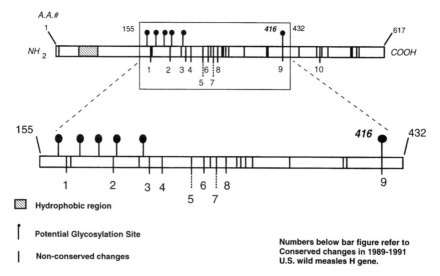

Figure 2   Diagram of the hemagglutinin protein of measles virus indicating regions of conservation and variation of the 1989–1991 U.S. wildtype strain relative to the vaccine strain hemagglutinin.

CD46, as a receptor for measles virus (Naniche et al., 1993) introduces at least one major bottleneck in the evolution of measles virus. Mutations that arise in measles variants that might affect pathogenicity or virulence, but are distinct from the hemagglutinin gene, would be lost if a critical change in the HA gene occurred that no longer permitted receptor binding. Thus, the changes in H coding region must be viewed as not interfering with receptor interaction and may only reflect the limited plasticity of the H molecule i.e., those areas that can undergo change without adversely affecting receptor binding function to CD46.

Cross-neutralization studies using vaccine viruses and representative wild-type viruses indicated that sera from recently infected individuals neutralize the current wild-type viruses 6 to 8 times better than they neutralized the vaccine strain. Serum specimens obtained from vaccinated individuals living outside measles virus endemic areas neutralized the vaccine and wild-type strains to essentially the same degree. One interpretation of these data is that the vaccine and wild-type viruses share common epitopes. Moreover, the wild-type must have at least one unique or sufficiently modified region on the H protein that is perhaps more immunodominant than that present on the vaccine strain. The H genes of both the U.S. vaccine strain and 1989 U.S. wild-type have been cloned into vaccinia expression vectors and were used to immunize both mice and rabbits. The relative difference in neutralization titers was maintained in these outbred animals, and the study clearly demonstrates that the neutralization differences are attributable to the antibody response to the H protein alone (Tamin et al., 1994).

While demonstrable changes in both the genetic and antigenic nature of the H protein are unquestionably present in some currently circulating wild-type viruses, such changes have not altered vaccine efficacy. The vaccine remains fully capable of eliciting an immune response that is protective against the current strains. The significance of the changes in H is not yet clear, but the findings do raise some relevant questions pertinent to the epidemiology, and control of measles virus with current vaccine strains.

Molecular epidemiology of measles virus

Although both genetic and antigenic changes could easily be demonstrated to have occurred between the wild measles virus circulating in the U.S. during the resurgent period and vaccine strains, no clear demonstration that such variation contributed to the resurgence of measles could be made. This period did provide a tremendous opportunity for the study of measles virus variability, and has led to the availability of a great number of nucleotide sequences of measles isolates from all over the world. It is now recognized that there are at least six different lineages of measles virus currently circulating worldwide (Rima et al., 1995a). Much of this analysis is based on the last 151 amino acids of the carboxyl terminus of the N gene, as well as the entire coding region of the H gene (Taylor et al., 1991). Regardless of the sequence used for analysis, measles virus strains examined separate into six or seven different genotypes, many of which

GENETIC GROUPS OF MEASLES VIRUS

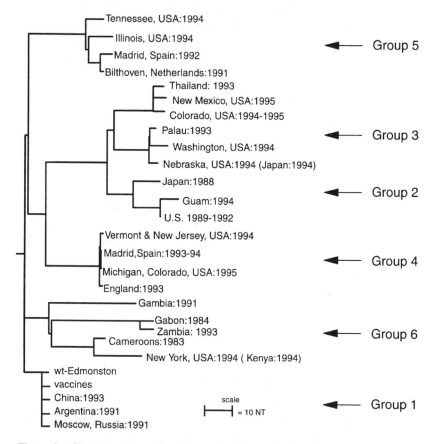

Figure 3   Genetic relationships of measles viruses isolated from recent outbreaks. Phenogram is based on the sequences of the H gene. Group 1 appears to
have had a very wide distribution during the pre-vaccine era and contains the
prototype Edmonston strain and all of the known vaccine strains. This group also
contains several wild-type viruses that were isolated in the U.S. and Europe in
the 1950s and 1960s. Wild-type viruses from group 1 have been isolated in Argentina, Russia and China in 1991–1993. Each of these strains has several unique
nucleotide substitutions in the H, N or F genes that differentiate them from the
vaccine strain or Edmonston so it is unlikely that they represent laboratory con-
taminants. Group 2 contains viruses that were associated with the resurgence of
measles cases in the U.S. between 1989 and 1991. Also, included in this diverse
group are recent isolates from Japan, China, Canada and Guam.

are depicted in Figure 3. (See Review by Rima et al., 1995b and Rota et al., 1994).

It is of interest to note that the fewest number of reported measles cases in the U.S. prior to the recent resurgence was in 1983. Although purely speculative, one interpretation of this result is that the 1983 lineage of virus may have been almost eliminated by the U.S. vaccination campaigns, only to be replaced by a strain that may have arisen in the United Kingdom.

With the molecular characterization of additional measles viruses isolated in the U.S. during 1989–1992, a consistent genotype was identified that apparently was the predominate genetic strain during the resurgent period. These wild-type isolates were genetically similar despite the patient's underlying medical conditions, source material for virus isolation, and the year and/or location of the outbreak or case. The dendrogram (Figure 4) reflects the near identity of these isolates with respect to the H gene sequence. This result suggested that this genotype was established in the susceptible population of the U.S. from the beginning of the resurgence and remained as the dominant indigenous strain throughout that period. In 1993, the fewest number of measles cases, 312, were reported. In conjunction with this historic low was a period of six weeks when no measles cases occurred that could not be linked to imported cases, and a three consecutive weeks period when no measles cases were reported by any county in the U.S. These data strongly suggested that indigenous transmission of measles was actually interrupted. Other factors that

---

(Figure 3, continued)

Groups 3 and 4 were defined very recently after analysis of viruses associated with outbreaks occurring between 1993 and 1995. Group 5 contains viruses from recent outbreaks that were related to a strain that was isolated in the U.S. in 1977. Viruses within group 6 show a high degree of genetic heterogeneity and these strains have been isolated in Africa or traced to direct importations from African countries. Aside from the African group (group 6), there appears to be no geographic restriction to the circulation of these contemporary genotypes of MV. Rather, it seems that multiple genotypes can co-circulate in any area.

**Dendrogram of Measles Virus isolates Based on H Sequence
Analysis from the U.S. Resurgent Period**

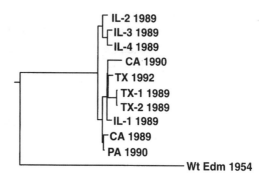

⊢——⊣ = 6 nucleotides

Figure 4   Genetic variation of MV within an epidemic. Phenogram shows the genetic relationships between the H genes of 10 wild-type MVs isolated during the resurgence of MV in the United States between 1988 and 1990. Recent isolates from Illinois (IL), California (CA), Texas (TX), and Pennsylvania (PA) were compared to a low passage seed of the Edmonston strain (wtEdm).

would have contributed to the break in transmission are the mass vaccination programs initiated in Mexico, Central and South America by the Pan American Health Organization (PAHO, 1994), and our own vaccine campaigns and two-dose schedules in response to the resurgence.

During 1994, measles cases numbered over one thousand, but their distribution reverted to that prior to the resurgent period. Cases occurred predominantly among high school- and college-aged persons, many of whom could provide evidence of one dose of vaccine. Over 45% of the spread cases occurred in religious or philosophically exempt groups, and many of the index cases could be traced to importations from outside the U.S. (CDC, 1994). Molecular epidemiology (nucleotide sequencing) both confirmed the imported nature of many of the index cases of measles, and provided further evidence that a break in the indigenous transmission of measles had occurred as suggested by the conventional epidemiology. Of the seven outbreaks in the U.S. from which measles isolates were obtained, none were the genotype of the dominant strain present during the resurgent period. In contrast, that genotype was isolated from specimens from a large outbreak (>200 cases) predominantly among preschool-aged children that occurred in Guam from February to June, 1994. These data suggest that mass vaccination campaigns launched at the time of the resurgence were successful in eliminating the dominant genotype of measles from the U.S. that was circulating during the resurgent period. New outbreaks (post 1993) did not involve that genotype, but instead seemed to consist of genotypes of measles that could be identified as circulating in other countries.

Molecular epidemiology could also be used to determine the path of transmission of virus from outbreak to outbreak. For example, an outbreak of measles among young adults at a Colorado ski resort extended into nine other states. One of the subsequent outbreaks resulted in 247 cases of measles in unvaccinated students of a religious exempt group attending college in Illinois or a school in St. Louis, Missouri. Coincident with the outbreak at the ski resort, a large outbreak of measles (>100 cases) was occurring at Rutgers University in New Jersey. That outbreak was started by a measles-infected student returning from Spain to Rutgers. Unfortunately the disease at Rutgers went undiagnosed for several infectious cycles before measles was recognized and control measures instituted. There were some anecdotal reports implying that measles-infected Rutgers students went to the ski resort for Spring Break.

The H gene genotypes of measles isolates from the Rutgers outbreak were determined to be distinctly different from those derived from Missouri and Illinois. The latter genotypes resembled one that was identified to have circulated in Western Europe. Of greater interest was the fact that a closely related genotype was involved in a small outbreak of measles in high school students in Tennessee. Although not confirmed by conventional epidemiology, molecular epidemiology indicated that the outbreaks of measles in Colorado, Missouri, and Illinois were not the result of poor control of the Rutgers outbreak, but instead may have been an extension of the Tennessee outbreak or independently fostered by an import from Western Europe (Rota et al., 1996).

Summary

Many lessons can be learned from the recent resurgence of measles disease in the U.S. We learned that insufficient vaccine coverage, particularly among the younger age groups in inner cities, will lead to the accumulation of enough susceptible individuals to maintain an outbreak. We learned that rapid spread of essentially a single genotype can occur between and among these susceptible communities. We also learned that it is possible that high vaccination rates can interrupt the transmission of measles. However, it is critical to maintain high levels of vaccine coverage even at apparent low points of activity to assure that there will not be sustained transmission of viruses introduced from other parts of the world. The present 2-dose schedule is designed to prevent the accumulation of susceptible individuals and to ensure that all persons receive at least 1 dose of vaccine (CDC, 1990).

The frequency of international air travel will hamper efforts to prevent continual re-introduction of measles virus into areas in which indigenous virus has been eliminated. It should also be noted that the unusually high infectious nature of measles virus may result in a very mixed pattern of genotypes across large geographical areas such as Europe for example (see Figure 3). However, the identification of circulating genotypes and the ability to recognize links between outbreaks will be beneficial in surveillance and formulation of strategies for measles control. If the interruption of transmission of indigenous measles can be achieved by use of measles vaccine, there can be hope for eradication of measles. However, until there is cooperation among all nations in the vaccination and surveillance for measles, the highly contagious nature of the virus will frustrate even the most aggressive programs.

Bibliography

Albrecht, P., Ennis, F. A., Salzman, F. J., and Krugman, S. (1977). Persistence of maternal antibody in infants beyond 12 months: mechanism of measles vaccine failure. *J. Pediatr.* *91*:915–918.

Atkinson, W. L., and Orenstein, W. A. (1992). The resurgence of measles in the United States, 1989–1990. *Ann. Rev. Med.* *43*:451–463.

Bromberg, K. M., Clark-Golden, M., Light, H., Shah, B., Marcellino, L., Rivera, M., Li,

P-W., Erdman, D., Heath, J., and Bellini, W. J. (1994). Maternal and infant immunity to measles. *J. Pediatr. 125*:579–581.

Centers for Disease Control. (1989). Measles—United States, first 26 weeks, 1989. *MMWR 38*:863–866.

Centers for Disease Control. (1990). Measles prevention: recommendations of the Immunization Practices Advisory Committee (ACIP). *MMWR 38 (No, S–9)*:1–18.

Centers for Disease Control. (1991). Measles vaccination levels among selected groups of preschool-aged children—United States. *MMWR 40*:305–306.

Centers of Disease Control. (1994). Measles—United States, first 26 weeks, 1994. *MMWR 43*:673–676.

Edmonson, M., Addiss, D., McPherson, J., Berg, J., Circo, S., Davis, J. (1990). Mild measles and secondary vaccine failure during a sustained outbreak in a highly vaccinated population. *JAMA 163*:2467–2471.

Ender, J. F., Peebles, T. C., McCarthy, K., Milovanovic, M., Mitus, A., Holloway, A. (1957). Measles virus: a summary of experiments concerned with isolation, properties, and behavior. *Am. J. Pub. Hth. 47*:275–282.

Erdman, D. D., Heath, J. L., Watson, J. C., Markowitz, L. E., and Bellini, W. J. (1993). Immunoglobulin M antibody response to measles virus following primary and secondary vaccination and natural infection. *J. Med. Virol. 41*:44–48.

Hummel, K. B., Erdman, D. D., Heath, J. L., and Bellini, W. J. (1992). Baculovirus expression of the nucleoprotein gene of measles virus and utility of the recombination protein in diagnostic enzyme immunoassays. *J. Clin. Microbiol. 30*:2874–2880.

Naniche, D., Varior-Krishnan, G., Cervoni, F., Wild, T. F., Rossi, B., Rabourdin-Combe, C., Gerlier, D. (1993). Human membrane cofactor protein (CD46) acts as a cellular receptor for measles virus. *J. Virol. 67*:6025–6032.

Pabst, H. F., Spady, D. W., Marusyk, R. G. (1992). Reduced measles immunity in infants in a well-vaccinated population. *Pediatr. Infect. Dis. 11*:525–529.

Pan American Health Organization (1994). Measles elimination by the year 2000. EPI Newsletter 16(5):1–2.

Rima, B. K., Earle, J. A. P., Yeo, R. P., Herlihy, L., Baczko, K., ter Meulen, V., Carabana, J., Caballero, M., Celma, M. L., and Fernandez-Munoz, R. (1995a). Temporal and geographical distribution of measles virus genotypes. *J. Gen. Virol. 76*:1173–1180.

Rima, B., Earle, J. A. P., Baczko, K., Rota, P. A., and Bellini, W. J. (1995b). *Measles Virus Strain Variations*. In: V. ter Meulen and M. Billeter, eds. Current Topics in Microbiology and Immunology. Measles Virus. Springer Verlag, Berlin-Heidelberg, pp. 65–83.

Rota, J. S., Hummel, K. B., Rota, P. A., Bellini, W. J. (1992). Genetic variability of the glycoprotein genes of current wild-type measles isolates. *Virology 188*:135–142.

Rota, J. S., Wang, Z–D., Rota, P. A., and Bellini, W. J. (1994a). Comparison of sequences of the H, F, and N coding genes of measles virus vaccine strains. *Virus Res. 31*:317–330.

Rota, P. A., Bloom, A. E., Vanchiere, J. A., and Bellini, W. J. (1994b). Evolution of the nucleoprotein and matrix genes of wild-type strains of measles virus isolated from recent epidemics. *Virology 198*:724–730.

Rota, J. S., Heath J. L., Rota, P. A., King, G. E., Celma, M. L., Carabana, J., Fernandez-Munoz, R., Brown, D., Jin, L., and Bellini, W. J. (1995). Molecular epidemiology of measles virus: Identification of pathways of transmission and the implications for measles elimination. *J. Inf. Dis. 173*:32–37.

Sakata, H., Kobune, F., Sato, T. A., Tanabayashi, K., Yamada, A., Sigiura, A. (1993). Variation in field isolates of measles virus during an 8-year period in Japan. *Microbiol. Immunol. 37*:233–237.

Tamin, A., Rota, P. A., Wang, Z., Heath, J., Anderson, L. J., and Bellini, W. J. (1994). Antigenic analysis of current wild-type and vaccine strains of measles virus. *J. Inf. Dis. 170*:795–801.

Taylor, M. J., Godfrey, E., Baczko, K., ter Meulen, V., Wild, T. F., and Rima, B. K. (1991). Identification of several different lineages of measles virus. *J. Gen. Virol. 72*:83–88.

8

Mechanisms of hepatitis B virus (HBV) persistence and associated disease

William S. Robinson, M.D.
Stanford University School of Medicine
Stanford, California 94305, USA

This review concerns some of the factors that are involved in persistence of hepatitis B virus and related hepadnaviruses, and mechanisms involved in different disease syndromes associated with persistent infection.

Hepadnaviruses

Hepadnaviridae (or hepadnaviruses) consist of a family of viruses that are closely related and have similar biological, molecular, and epidemiologic features, and are associated with similar disease syndromes including hepatocellular carcinoma (HCC). The family name (*Hepadnaviridae*) indicates the DNA genome and hepatotropism of these viruses (1–3). The hepadnavirus family includes hepatitis B virus (HBV) of man, woodchuck hepatitis virus (WBV) of *Marmata monax* (4), ground squirrel hepatitis virus (GSHV) of *Spermophilus beecheyi* (5), duck hepatitis B virus (DHBV) found in several varieties of domestic ducks (6) and similar viruses in tree squirrels (7), and herons (8). Less well documented findings in other rodents, marsupials, and cats suggest that other hepadnaviruses may exist.

Common features of hepadnaviruses include virion (virus particle) size and ultrastructure with an envelope surrounding an electron dense spherical nucleocapsid or core; characteristic polypeptide and antigenic composition; common virion DNA size, structure, and genetic organization; the presence of DNA polymerase (reverse transcriptase) activity in the virion; and an unusual mechanism of viral DNA replication which includes reverse transcription of a greater than genome length viral RNA transcript of the viral DNA genome (reviewed in 9). Hepadnaviruses have regions of DNA sequence homology with retroviruses and cauliflower mosaic virus; share features of gene number, function and organization; and all utilize a reverse transcriptase mechanism in viral genome replication (10, 11). Characteristic features of these viruses include hepatic tropism, a propensity to cause persistent infection under some circumstances, and the presence of high concentrations of viral forms in the blood of almost all infected individuals. In common with other blood-borne viruses, HBV is transmitted by sexual contacts, by percutaneous exposure to blood and from infected mothers to newborn and/or young children.

Structure of the viral genome

The DNA genome of these viruses (reviewed in 9) is among the smallest of all known animal viruses consisting of an approximately 3200 base pair circular molecule that contains a single stranded region of different length in different molecules (see Fig. 1) reflecting the fact that DNA molecules are packaged into virions before viral DNA replication (i.e. synthesis of the DNA plus strand) is complete (see virus replication below). The virion DNA strands are not closed circular molecules but each is discontinuous with a 5′ end at a unique nucleotide sequence position as shown in Fig. 1. The overlapping cohesive 5′ ends of the two DNA strands hold the double stranded DNA in a circular conformation.

The genomes of the 3 mammalian hepadnaviruses have 4 long open reading frames in the complete or long (minus) virion DNA strand and these have similar locations in each virus with respect to the cohesive ends of the virion DNA (Fig. 1). These encode the viral polypeptides of : 1) the viral envelope which contain hepatitis B surface antigen (HBsAg) specificity, 2) the viral nucleocapsid or core which contains hepatitis B core antigen (HBcAg) specificity and the soluble protein which is a truncated form of the major core protein and manifests hepatitis Be antigen

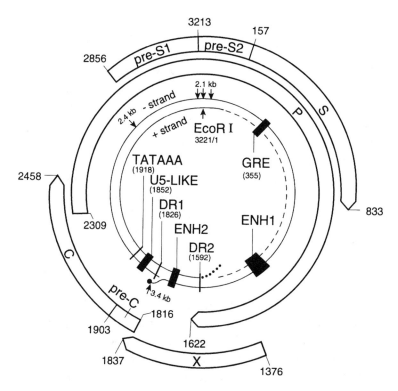

Figure 1 Circular map of the HBV (adw2) genome. The inner circles represent the virion DNA strands and the broken (dashed) line in the short (+) DNA strand represents the region within which the 3' end of the + strand may occur in different molecules, and the corresponding region of the long strand is that which may be single-stranded in different molecules. A line of dots represents the oligoribonucleotide primer covalently attached to the 5' end of the + DNA strand and a single dot represents the protein primer covalently attached to the 5' end of the—DNA strand. The large arrows represent the recognized functional open reading frames (ORF) with the direction of transcription from the minus DNA strand 10 indicated. The small arrows indicate the 5'-ends of the three A major size classes of transcripts of 3.4, 2.4 and 2.1 Kb, all of which are identically terminated near the poly A addition signal (TATAAA). The nucleotide sequence locations of the initiation and termination codons of each ORF are given with reference to map position 1 at the single EcoRI cleavage site in this DNA. The map position of the first nucleotide of the glucocorticoid responsive element (GRE), DR2, DR1, the U5-like sequence and the poly A addition sequence (TATAAA) are indicated, as are the general regions exhibiting enhancer 1 (ENH 1) and enhancer 2 (ENH 2) activity.

(HBeAg) specificity, 3) the largest polypeptide which has reverse transcriptase activity, RNAse H activity and is the protein primer for synthesis of the viral minus DNA strand, and 4) the small X protein which has the capacity to transactivate transcription regulated by both homologous and heterologous regulatory elements. Hepadnaviruses do not encode an integrase protein like that of retroviruses which facilitates viral genome integration.

Other functionally important elements in hepadnavirus genomes (reviewed in 9) include two 11 bp direct repeat sequences designated DR1 and DR2 (involved in viral DNA replication) which are approximately 225 bp apart in the mammalian viruses respectively located at genome sequence positions near the 5' ends of virion DNA. Four promoter elements for transcription, three transcriptional enhancer elements (enhancers 1 and 2, and a glucocorticoid responsive enhancer element), and a polyadenylation signal used by all major transcripts lies within the beginning of the C–gene.

The hepadnavirus genome is unusually compact and efficiently organized in that much of the genome is utilized for multiple functions including overlapping genes so that the same nucleotide sequence encodes more than one protein and all cis–acting regulatory sequences (e.g. transcriptional enhancer and promoter elements) are contained in genomic sequences also encoding protein (see Fig. 1).

Viral genome replication and integration

Replication of the viral genome (Fig. 2) involves conversion of infecting virion DNA molecules into covalently closed circular molecules in liver cell nuclei; formation of a greater than genome length RNA transcript with a terminally-repeated sequence and shorter transcripts which function as messenger RNAs; packaging of the long transcript, newly-made viral reverse transcriptase and protein primer in viral core particles found in hepatocyte cytoplasm; and synthesis of new viral DNA molecules by reverse transcription of the long RNA transcript utilizing a viral encoded protein primer in forming the first synthesized viral DNA (minus) strand and a capped oligoribonucleotide derived from the 5' end of the long RNA template as primer for synthesis of the second DNA (plus) strand,

Hepadnavirus Replication

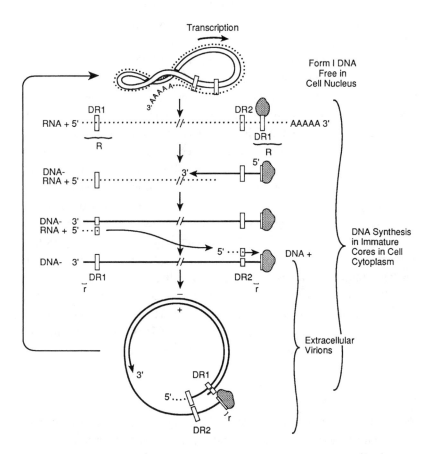

Figure 2   Scheme of proposed mechanism of hepadnavirus DNA replication. DR–1 and DR–2 represent 11 nucleotide pair direct repeat sequences. R represents the approximately 200 nucleotide terminal redundancy in the long RNA transcript and r represents the short terminal redundancy of the minus DNA strand. Solid lines represent DNA strands, dotted lines RNA and the stippled area the protein primer for DNA strand synthesis.

exclusively within cytoplasmic viral core particles (reviewed in 12–14). There is a nine nucleotide terminal redundancy in the minus-strand which may function in strand switching by the DNA polymerase during viral DNA replication.

Ordered integration of viral DNA in cellular DNA is not an intrinsic part of hepadnavirus replication as it is for replication of retroviruses. However, sporadic viral integration by a mechanism such as illegitimate recombination does take place and integrated viral DNA has been found in cellular DNA of infected liver as well as hepatocellular carcinoma (reviewed in 15 and 16). In hepadnavirus infected hosts, many HCC contain viral integrations with a clonal pattern. It follows that these tumors must have arisen by clonal expansion of an original cell with that viral integration. The possible role of such integrations in development of HCC has been intensively investigated (see Section 6). Much of the evidence of the fine structure of hepadnavirus integrations comes from investigation of those in human (reviewed in 17–19) and woodchuck (20) HCCs; there has been much less investigation of viral integrations in non–tumorous liver. It is not known whether viral integration occurs in every hepadnavirus infected cell *in vivo* or only in some cells. However, no apparent difference in the structure of viral integrations of HCC and non–tumorous liver have been identified.

Viral forms in the blood

Viral forms that are present in the blood of infected individuals (reviewed in 9) include multiple morphological forms of the viral surface antigen (Fig. 3). The most numerous is a small spherical 20 nanometer form and filamentous forms without nucleocapsid (core) protein or viral DNA. Virions with a surface antigen containing envelope and internal nucleocapsid with the viral core antigen, viral DNA and viral DNA polymerase (reverse transcriptase) are present in blood at lower concentrations. Viral e antigen in the blood is a truncated form of the viral core polypeptide that is secreted by infected cells with replicating virus and appears in an extracellular form as a soluble antigen. The viral core and e antigens share amino acid sequence and T-cell epitopes but have different antibody specificities (B cell epitopes).

HEPATITIS B VIRUS ANTIGEN FORMS IN THE BLOOD

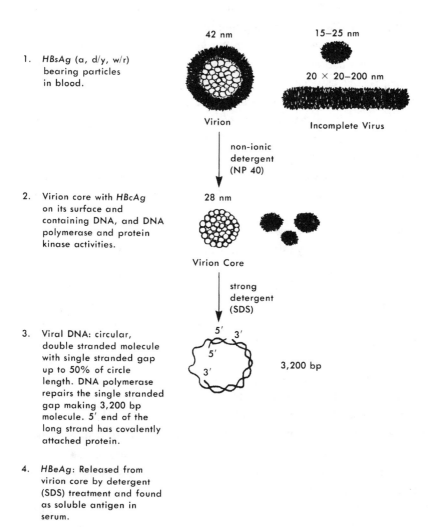

1. *HBsAg* (a, d/y, w/r) bearing particles in blood.

2. Virion core with *HBcAg* on its surface and containing DNA, and DNA polymerase and protein kinase activities.

3. Viral DNA: circular, double stranded molecule with single stranded gap up to 50% of circle length. DNA polymerase repairs the single stranded gap making 3,200 bp molecule. 5' end of the long strand has covalently attached protein.

4. *HBeAg*: Released from virion core by detergent (SDS) treatment and found as soluble antigen in serum.

Figure 3   Schematic representation of hepatitis B viral forms found in the blood of infected patients.

Factors that promote viral persistence

Viral persistence is a common outcome of hepadnavirus infection and such persistent infections commonly last for the remaining lifetime of the individual. HBV infections commonly occur at early ages and become persistent in populations in which this virus is highly endemic such as in eastern Asia and sub-Saharan Africa (21). Such persistent HBV infections may be associated with chronic hepatitis. Viral surface antigen (HBsAg) particles can be detected in the blood of almost all persistently infected individuals and virions, infectious virus and e antigen (HBeAg) are present in many. Persistent infection is usually defined as serum HBsAg positivity for 6 months or more. With time HBsAg titers fall; and HBeAg, virions and infectious virus fall below detectable levels in the serum of many patients with chronic HBV infection and persisting serum HBsAg.

Several factors have been identified that influence virus persistence including age of primary infection, infecting dose of virus, immunocompetence of the host, sex of the host, and possibly other genetic and/or environmental factors. The most dramatic effect is caused by age of primary infection. Primary HBV infection of adults has been shown to result in persistent infection (HBsAg persisting in serum for 6 months or more) in less than 1% to 10% of cases in different studies (22–26). The remaining patients have self-limited infections with markers of active HBV infection such as serum HBsAg becoming undetectable within a few days or weeks. In contrast, primary HBV infection has been shown to result in persistence in 90% to 95% of newborn infants (27–30) and approximately 20% of preschool children (31). This dramatic effect of age of primary infection on viral persistence is also observed in the animal models (woodchucks, Beechey ground squirrels and ducks) with the respective natural virus of each host.

A second factor that appears to influence persistence of these viruses is the infecting dose of virus. In a single study carried out in the early 1950s (32) in which defined doses of HBV (serial dilutions of an HBsAg positive serum) were each inoculated into several human volunteers it was demonstrated that the lower the infecting dose of virus the shorter the incubation period, the milder the initial disease (acute hepatitis) and the

Table 8.1. *Three mammalian hosts in which chronic hepadnavirus infection is associated with HCC*

Host (age of infection)	Time of infection to first HCC	HCC "Incidence" in infected host
Woodchuck (WHV infection at birth) (ref. 52, 53)	< 1 yr	100% in 2 yrs
Beechey ground squirrel (GSHV infection at birth) (ref. 55)	4.5 yrs	67% in 6.5 yrs
Human [HBV infection, 1/3 at birth and others at young age] (ref. 49)	~30 yrs*	40% lifetime risk for HBsAg+ middle aged Chinese males.

*HBV associated HCCs occur infrequently before age 30 yrs.

higher the probability of viral persistence beyond 6 months. A similar study in chimpanzees confirmed the relationship of virus dose to incubation period but not to persistent infection (33).

A third factor that influences the course of hepadnavirus infection is immunosuppression. Patients with persistent HBV infection are not immunologically tolerant to the virus in that they have antibody responses to viral antigens during persistent infection. All have very high antibody responses to core antigen that persists throughout infection, and many such patients continuously produce antibody to surface antigen that can be detected in serum antigen–antibody complexes. Most patients develop antibody responses to e antigen at the time HBeAg becomes undetectable in the blood (HBeAg to anti-HBe seroconversion). HLA restricted cytotoxic T cell responses directed at cells expressing viral antigens have been demonstrated in some patients with chronic HBV infection and most such cases have significant chronic hepatitis (34, 35). Thus, persistently infected patients are not immunologically tolerant to viral antigens. However, anecdotal evidence indicates that renal transplant patients and other immunocompromised patients are more likely to have mild disease after hepatitis B virus infection and the infection becomes persistent more often than in immunologically normal adults (e.g. 36, 37). Immunosuppressive therapy of HBsAg carriers results in evidence of increased virus replication with a rise in titers of serum HBsAg, HBeAg and virions and a higher fraction of cells with detectable viral antigen in liver biopsies. Glucocorticoid therapy may also enhance virus replication by activating a glucocorticoid responsive transcriptional enhancer element in the viral genome (38).

A fourth factor that appears to influence hepadnavirus persistence is the sex of the host. Studies of HBsAg prevalence in many but not all populations has shown that the prevalence of the carrier state is higher in males than females (39, 40). The cause of that sex difference is not understood. The rate of persistence appears to be the same in both sexes following neonatal infection in populations in which most infections occur at very young ages suggesting that the difference in prevalence found at older ages in those populations may be due to more frequent resolution of persistent infection in females than in males. No sex difference in persistent infection rates has been observed in hepadnavirus infected woodchucks, ground squirrels or ducks.

Finally, there has been much interest in identifying other genetic and/or environmental factors that influence persistent infection to account for the dramatic differences in persistent HBV infection in different populations around the world. For example, in some South Pacific islands populations the prevalence of serum HBsAg is up to 25%, and in China and some other Asian and sub-Saharan African populations carrier rates around 10% are found (21). In contrast in the U.S. and Northern European countries carrier rates are closer to 0.1%. Whether these differences are due to genetic factors that predispose individuals to persistent infection in some populations, to different cultural factors that promote virus transmission at early ages in some populations or to other mechanisms is not clear. There has been no consistent correlation of rates of virus persistence with genetic markers such as HLA types.

A common feature among the above described conditions that appear to increase the chance of viral persistence may be that each impairs or alters the immune response to virus infection in such a way that precludes elimination of the virus, although clearly persistently infected hosts are not immunologically tolerant to the virus.

Pathogenetic mechanisms of hepadnavirus-associated disease

Hepadnavirus infections can be associated with several different disease syndromes that result from different pathogenetic mechanisms. One is necroinflammatory liver disease in the form of acute or chronic hepatitis B. Liver injury with liver cell necrosis, and host responses including inflammation, lymphocytic infiltration, and liver regeneration are prominent parts of this disease process. Macronodular cirrhosis develops in a significant fraction of persistently HBV infected humans, usually after many years (21,41). The most widely accepted concept is that liver cell necrosis results from immunologic injury directed at viral antigens in infected liver cells. An HLA class I-restricted cytotoxic T-cell (CTL) response directed at hepatitis B core (HBcAg) and e (HBeAg) antigens has most often been implicated (34, 35). On the other hand it has not been easy to demonstrate antigen specific CTL and such CTL when detected in peripheral blood or liver have been found in very low numbers in patients with acute or chronic hepatitis B (35). Thus, other immunological and nonimmunologic mechanisms for liver cell necrosis must also be considered. There is experimental evidence suggesting two possible non-immunological mechanisms for liver cell injury. One is HBcAg expression that has been shown to be cytotoxic to cells in culture (42). A second is that overexpression of the large hepatitis B surface antigen protein and its accumulation in liver cells because it is not secreted leads to liver cell necrosis and hepatitis in transgenic mice (43). Whether either of these mechanisms leads to liver cell injury associated with natural hepadnavirus infection in humans or animals is unclear but deserves further study.

A different pathogenetic mechanism resulting in different disease syndromes in hepadnavirus infection is immune complex-mediated disease.

Hepatitis B surface antigen–antibody complexes have been implicated in the serum sickness-like prodromal illness that is seen in 15% of patients with acute hepatitis B, with rash, sometimes urticaria, arthralgia, arthritis and fever (44, 45). Necrotizing arteritis or polyarteritis, seen in a small number of HBV infected patients following acute hepatitis B that becomes persistent is associated with HBsAg-anti-HBS immune complexes and complement in the walls of involved arteries (reviewed in 46, 47). Similarly, glomerulonephritis following acute hepatitis B is associated with similar immune complexes and complement in glomerular basement membranes (reviewed in 46, 47).

A disease that is associated with persistent hepadnavirus infection and undoubtedly results from a still different pathogenetic mechanism is liver cancer (reviewed in 15, 16 and 48). Long-standing HBV infection is associated with a greatly increased risk of hepatocellular carcinoma (HCC) compared with the risk in uninfected populations (21, 49–51), and the presence of cirrhosis in HBV-infected individuals appears to further increase the risk of HCC by at least ten-fold (49). The association of persistent hepadnavirus infection with HCC is even stronger for WHV infected woodchucks (52,53) and GSHV infected Beechey ground squirrels (54, 55) (Table 1). Although the importance of infection with these viruses in development of HCC is clear, the mechanism by which the viruses act is not as clear. Interestingly, a different potentially oncogenic genetic change has been found at a significant frequency (e.g. >25%) in HCC of each of these mammalian hosts, and a fourth potentially oncogenic mechanism has been identified which could be important for hepadnavirus-associated HCC in all three hosts. Two of the genetic alterations result from a specific viral effect and the other two appear to be unrelated to a specific viral mechanism.

One viral specific genetic change found in HCC is viral insertional mutagenesis. Most HCCs of hepadnavirus infected hosts contain integrated viral sequences in host DNA (reviewed in 15–18, 48, 56) and this has long raised the question of whether such integrations ever contribute to oncogenesis. However, the hepatitis B viral integrations that have been extensively investigated in human HCC have all been found at different cellular genomic sites and no unique cellular DNA site for viral integration has been found (17, 18, 57). Very few HBV integrations have been found near or within any cellular gene and most are within noncoding repetitive cellular DNA sequences (17, 18). An oncogenic effect of the integrations in the few human HCCs in which viral integrants were found near or within cellular genes (58, 59) remains unproven. Thus viral insertional mutagenesis appears to be excluded as a common oncogenic mechanism in the case of HBV in human HCC.

More recently, however, strong evidence has been obtained for viral insertional mutagenesis which results in cis–activation of the expression of certain oncogenes in a significant number of HCC of WHV infected woodchucks. WHV integrations near c-myc (60–62) and N-myc (63–65) genes have been found in up to 50% of woodchuck HCC and transcriptional regulatory elements of the integrated viral sequences appear to activate expression of the respective cellular gene in the cases studied (60–63). The high prevalence of WHV integrations which cis–activate c-myc or N-myc genes in woodchuck HCCs suggests that viral integrations at these sites is not incidental in this system but they are probably selected in HCC because of their oncogenic effects. Viral integrations near N-myc or c-myc have not been reported in human (17, 18, 64, 65) or ground squirrel (66) HCCs suggesting that this mechanism is common for WHV in woodchuck HCC but not for GSHV in ground squirrel HCC or HBV in human HCC. A recent study (67) comparing HCC in WHV infected woodchucks and GSHV infected woodchucks revealed evidence for WHV integration near the N-myc gene in 7 of 17 woodchuck HCC (confirming the previous findings). In contrast, in GSHV infected woodchucks evidence for GSHV integration near N-myc was found in only 1 of 16 HCC suggesting that viral integration at this site is more common for WHV than for GSHV in HCC of woodchucks infected with the different respective viruses.

A second potentially oncogenic genetic alteration, c-myc gene amplification and over-expression, has been found in 6 of 14 HCC of Beechey ground squirrels (66). This high prevalence of c-myc amplification suggests a significant relationship of this change with HCC in this host. However, it is not clear whether this change is an early event that plays a role in initiating HCC or is a secondary change arising during tumor growth. There is no evidence that GSHV plays a role in c-myc amplification since it has been found in HCC of animals without active GSHV infection as well as in actively infected animals. C-myc amplification has not been reported in HCC of woodchucks (66) and appears rarely in human HCC (90) suggesting this change occurs commonly in ground squirrel HCC and not in HCC of the other two hosts.

A third potentially oncogenic genetic alteration is point mutations in and/or allelic deletions of the tumor suppressor gene p53 found in many human HCC. Nucleotide sequence analysis of p53 exons 5 to 8 has revealed p53 mutations in 8 of 16 human HCC from Qidong province of China (91) and 5 of 10 human HCC from South Africa (92). Sixteen of the mutations in these studies involved codon 249 (G to T and G to C transversions both resulting in a change in coding of arginine to serine). Other studies have revealed point mutations at other sites (and not in codon 249) of p53 (93) or have found no mutations in the p53 gene of HCC (94). It has been suggested that the occurrence of such point mutations may correlate with dietary aflatoxin B1 (95), a mycotoxin known to cause such transversions in DNA. Recent studies of the p53 gene in HCC of other hosts has revealed no mutation in the p53 gene of HCC of 14 ground squirrels and 11 woodchucks with ongoing or past hepadnavirus infection (96). A single point mutation (G to T changing cysteine codon to phenyl alanine) was found in exon 5 of the p53 gene of one of 6 HCC arising in ground squirrels treated with aflatoxin B1. This suggests that point mutations in the p53 gene are common in human HCC and not common in HCC of woodchucks or ground squirrels. Whether such mutations in human HCC are caused by aflatoxin B1 remains unproven but the finding of one such mutation in an HCC of one of six aflatoxin B1 treated ground squirrels (and none in those untreated) is consistent with this.

The p53 gene is on human chromosome 19p13 and loss of one allele of the p53 gene was found in 6 of 10 (97) and 5 of 8 (91) HCC respectively in two studies of human cases from China, in 3 of 5 HCC from southern Africa (92) and 12 of 33 from Japan (98). Deletions and rearrangements of the p53 gene have also been reported in some HCC cell lines (99) and altered expression of p53 was found in cell lines without deletion of the gene (99). There is no evidence that the point mutations found in the p53 gene of human HCC or allelic deletions are directly caused by HBV and all HCC in which these changes have been found are not from HBV infected hosts. It is not clear by what viral mechanism such changes could arise. Whether these changes are a factor in initiating HCC or are secondary changes arising during the growth of HCC remains undetermined.

A fourth mechanism with hepatocarcinogenic potential for all three hepadnavirus infected hosts is transactivation of cellular genes by a viral gene product. Mammalian hepadnaviruses do not contain a rapidly transforming gene such as the viral oncogenes of some retroviruses and certain DNA viruses since HBV appears to replicate in liver cells for many years without the occurrence of HCC. Hepadnaviruses do, however, contain a gene (designated the x gene) which encodes a transcriptional trans-activator protein capable of activating homologous and heterologous regulatory sequences (68, 69). The HBV X (hbx) protein has been shown to activate transcription controlled by regulatory sequences of the human beta–interferon gene (68), human immunodeficiency virus type 1 (HIV–1) (69–71), and simian virus 40 (SV40) (69, 72–74) [all of which contain a common DNA motif known as a kB site (a binding sequence for the nuclear transcription factor NF–kB) which has been shown to be an x-protein responsive element (73, 75)], the c-myc gene promoter (76, 77), c-jun regulatory sequences (78), the Rous sarcoma virus LTR (74, 79), and AP2 binding sequences (80), and HBV regulatory sequences (71, 72) [none of the latter contain a kB sequence]. Genes shown to be activated by hbx when expressed in cells include β-interferon (68), HIV (73), class I major histocompatibility complex gene (81), and the c-myc gene (76, 77). The different number of hbx responsive transcription regulatory elements, the failure to demonstrate hbx protein binding to any DNA sequence (79, 82) and the cell specificity of the hbx transactivation effect (83) suggest that a direct sequence specific interaction of hbx protein with DNA is not involved but transactivation is probably mediated through an effect on cellular transcription factors.

Partially transformed cell lines (76, 84) were rendered tumorigenic by hbx but primary cells in culture are not. HCC developed at 9 to 12 months of age in transgenic mice with liver specific expression of hbx (85). In addition, hbx has been detected in some human HCC with HBV integrations and the expressed X protein appears to have transcriptional transactivating activity (86, 87). These findings raise the possibility that hbx expression could contribute to hepatocarcinogenesis possibly by activating certain cellular genes. The evidence that hbx can activate the protooncogenes c-jun (78) and c-myc (76, 77), and that these genes are over-expressed in HCC of hepadnavirus infected hosts (78) is consistent with this.

Another HBV gene product that has been reported to transactivate transcription of heterologous genes is a truncated form of the pre S2/S gene product (88, 89). The number or fraction of HCC that express a truncated preS/S protein with transcriptional transactivating activity is not known and thus a possible role of such a mechanism in HCC is not defined.

Although transactivation of cellular genes by a viral gene product such as hbx is not at this time a proven viral mechanism in the pathogenesis of HCC, the evidence supporting this possibility is sufficient that this mechanism deserves further investigation.

A number of different additional genetic alterations including chromosomal translocations (100, 101), mutations in the N-ras gene (102) and other genes (103–105) and other changes have been found in isolated human HCCs or at a low frequency in human HCCs and not at a high frequency as are the four genetic changes described above (e.g. >25% in HCC of at least one host). Genetic events that occur rarely in HCC may contribute to hepatocarcinogenesis in individual HCC in which they are found but would appear not to represent a common or general mechanism in HCC.

Since a specific viral oncogenic mechanism has not been identified in most hepadnavirus associated HCC, there must be an as yet unidentified mechanism and some of these may be non-viral specific mechanisms that result in potentially oncogenic genetic changes in liver of HBV infected (and uninfected) humans. Supporting this possibility is that several different important risk factors for HCC (reviewed in 15, 16 and 48) including chronic hepatitis B, chronic hepatitis C, hemochromatosis, cryptogenic cirrhosis, biliary cirrhosis, autoimmune hepatitis and certain other factors which may cause cirrhosis all result in the common pathologic process of hepatocellular necrosis, inflammation and liver regeneration (necroinflammatory liver disease). This common pathologic process when continuing for a long period of time appears to be hepatocarcinogenic and the carcinogenic mechanism does not appear to depend on which of many diverse factors initiates the process of liver injury. It must be considered that chronic hepadnavirus infection could act through such a nonvirus specific mechanism (a chronic liver injury-response mechanism) and not cause HCC by a specific viral mechanism in many cases.

In conclusion, different potentially oncogenic genetic changes have been found at a significant frequency in HCC of different species (or associated with different hepadnaviruses) suggesting that hepatocarcinogenic mechanisms may be different in different species (or when arising in association with infection with different hepadnaviruses).

Some potentially oncogenic genetic changes found at a significant frequency in HCC of hepadnavirus infected hosts represent direct virus effects (viral enhancer insertion and cis–activation of c-myc and N-myc gene, and transactivation of cell genes by hbx) and others appear not to be caused by a direct viral mechanism (e.g. p53 gene mutation and c-myc gene amplification). Thus genetic events not resulting from direct effects of an hepadnavirus may be important in hepatocarcinogenesis in hepadnavirus infected hosts.

A causal or initiating effect of any genetic change in hepatocarcinogenesis is difficult to prove and distinguish from a secondary change arising during HCC growth and progression. The possibility of a causal role is strongest for WHV enhancer insertion which results in cis–activation of c-myc and N-myc genes.

In most tumor systems multiple genetic changes are required for full expression of the malignant phenotype (106–108). None of the changes found so far in HCC may be sufficient to cause HCC but one or more may represent contributing events.

Certain potentially oncogenic genetic changes that have been found infrequently in HCC of some animal species (e.g. viral insertional mutagenesis in human HCC) may contribute to pathogenesis of HCC in these specific cases but do not appear to represent a common or general mechanism in that species.

References

1. Robinson, W. S. (1980). Genetic variation among hepatitis B and related viruses. *Ann. New York Acad. Sci.* *354*:371–378.
2. Robinson, W. S., Marion, P. L., Feitelson, M. and Siddiqui, A. (1982). The hepadna virus group: hepatitis B and related viruses. In: Szmuness, W., Alter, H. J. and J. E. Maynard, (Eds.) *Viral Hepatitis.* Philadelphia: Franklin Institute Press; 57–68.

3. Gust, I. D., Burrell. C. J., Couplis, A. G., Robinson, W. S. and Zuckerman, A. J. (1986). Taxonomic classification of human hepatitis B virus. *Intervirology* 25:14–29.

4. Summers, J., Smolec, J. M., and Snyder, R. (1978). A virus similar to human hepatitis B virus associated with hepatitis and hepatoma in woodchucks. *Proc. Natl. Acad. Sci. USA* 75:4533–4537.

5. Marion, P. L., Oshiro, L., Regnery, D. C., Scullard, G. H., and Robinson, W. S. (1980). A virus in Beechey ground squirrels that is related to hepatitis B virus of man. *Proc. Natl. Acad. Sci. USA* 77:2941–2945.

6. Mason, W. S., Seal, G., Summers, J. (1980). Virus of Pekin ducks with structural and biological relatedness to human hepatitis B virus. *J. Virol.* 36:829–836.

7. Feitelson, M., Millman, I., and Blumberg, R. (1986). The hepadnavirus family: Animal Hepadnaviruses. *Proc. Natl. Acad. Sci. USA* 83:2994–2997.

8. Sprengel, R., Kaleta, E. F. and Will, H. (1988). Isolation and characterization of a hepatitis B virus endemic in herons. *J. Virol.* 62:3832–3839.

9. Robinson, W. S. (1990). Hepadnaviridae and their replication. In *Virology*, ed. B. Fields and D. M. Knipe, Raven Press, New York, pp. 2137–2169.

10. Toh, H., Hayashida, H., and Miyata, T. (1983). Sequence homology between retroviral reverse transcriptase and putative polymerases of hepatitis B virus and cauliflower mosaic virus. *Nature* 305:827–829.

11. Miller, R. H., Robinson, W. S. (1986). Common evolutionary origin of hepatitis B virus and retroviruses. *Proc. Natl. Acad. Sci. USA* 83:2531–2535.

12. Summers, J. and Mason, W. S. (1982). Replication of the genome of a hepatitis B-like virus by reverse transcription of an RNA intermediate. *Cell* 29:403–415.

13. Seeger, C., Ganem, D., and Varmus, H. E. (1986). Biochemical and genetic evidence for the hepatitis B virus replication strategy. *Science* 232:477.

14. Will, H., Reiser, W., Weimer, T., Pfaff, E., Buscher, M., Spreugal, R., Cattaneo, R., and Schaller, H. (1987). Replication strategy of human hepatitis B virus. *J. Virol.* 61:904–911.

15. Robinson, W. S. (1992). The role of hepatitis B virus in the development of primary hepatocellular carcinoma. Part. I. *J. Gast. Hep.* 7:622–638.

16. Robinson, W. S. (1993). The role of hepatitis B virus in development of primary hepatocellular carcinoma: Part II. *J. Gast. Hep.*8:95–106.

17. Nagaya, T., Nakamura, T., Tokino, T., Tsurimoto, T., Imai, M., Mayumi, T., Kamino, K., Yamamura, K. and Matsubara, K. (1987). The mode of hepatitis B virus DNA integration in chromosomes of human hepatocellular carcinoma. *Genes Dev.* 1:773–782.

18. Matsubara, K., Tokina, T. (1990). Integration of hepatitis B virus DNA and its implications for hepatocarcinogenesis. *Mol. Biol. Med.* 7:243–260.

19. Shih, C., Burke, K., Chou, M. J., Zeldis, J. B., Yang, C. S., Lee, C. S., Isselbacher, K. J., Wands, J. R. and Goodman, H. M. (1987). Tight clustering of human hepatitis B virus integration sites in hepatomas near a triple-stranded region. *J. Virol.* 61:3491–3498.

20. Ogston, C. W., Jonak, G. J., Rogler, C. E., Astrin, S. M. and Summers, J. (1982). Cloning and structural analysis of integrated woodchuck hepatitis virus sequences from hepatocellular carcinomas of woodchucks. *Cell 29*:385–394.

21. Szmuness, W. (1978). Hepatocellular carcinoma and the hepatitis B virus: evidence for a causal association. *Prog. Med. Virol. 24*:40–69.

22. Hoofnagle, J. H., Seeff, L. B., Bales, Z. B., Gerety, R. J., and Tabor, E. (1978). Serologic responses in hepatitis B. In: Vyas, G. N., Cohen, S. N., Schmid, R. (eds). *Viral Hepatitis: A Contemporary Assessment of Etiology. Epidemiology Pathogenesis and Prevention*. Philadelphia: Franklin Institute Press, pp. 219–242.

23. Redeker, A. G. (1975). Viral hepatitis: Clinical aspects. *Am. J. Med. Sci. 270*:9.

24. Seeff, L. B., Beebe, G. W., Hoofnagle, J. H., et al. (1987). A serologic follow-up of the 1942 epidemic of post-vaccination hepatitis in the U.S. Army. *New Engl. J. Med. 316*:965–970.

25. Norman, J. E., Beebe, G. W., Hoofnagle, J., Seeff, L. B. (1993). Mortality followup of the 1942 epidemic of hepatitis B in the U.S. Army. *Hepatology 18*:790–797.

26. Beasley, R. P., Hwang, L.-Y., Lin, C.-C., Ko, Y.-C., Twu, S. -J. (1983). Incidence of hepatitis among students at a university in Taiwan. *Am. J. Epidemiol. 117*:213–222.

27. Schweitzer, I. L., Dunn, A. E. F., Peters, R. L. and Spears, R. L. (1973). Viral hepatitis in neonates and infants. *Am. J. Med. 55*:762.

28. Tong, M. J., Thursby, M., Rakela, J., McPeak, C., Edwards, V. M. and Mosley, J. W. (1981). Studies of the maternal–infant transmission of the viruses which cause acute hepatitis. *Gastroenterology 80*:999.

29. Beasley, R. P., Hwang, L.-Y., Lin, C.-C., et al. (1981). Hepatitis B immune globulin (HBIG) efficacy in the interruption of perinatal transmission of hepatitis B virus carrier state. *Lancet 2*:388–393.

30. McMahon, B. J., Alward, W. L. M., Hall, D. B., et al. (1985). Acute hepatitis B virus infection: relation of age to the clinical expression of disease and subsequent development of the carrier state. *J. Infect. Dis. 151*:599–603.

31. Beasley, R. P., Hwang, L.-Y., Lin, C. -C., Ko, Y.-C., Twu, S.-J. (1982). Incidence of hepatitis B virus infections in preschool children in Taiwan. *J. Infect. Dis. 146*:198–204.

32. Barker, L. F., and Murray, R. (1972). Relationship of virus dose of incubation time of clinical hepatitis and time of appearance of hepatitis–associated antigen. *Am. J. Med. Sci. 263*:27.

33. Barker, L. F., Maynard, J. E., Purcell, R. H., et al. (1975). Hepatitis B virus infection in chimpanzees: titration of subtypes. *J. Infect. Dis. 132*:451–458.

34. Naumov, N. W., Mondelli M., Alexander, G. J. M., et al. (1984). Relationship between expression of hepatitis B virus antigens in isolated hepatocytes and autologous lymphocyte cytotoxicity in patients with chronic hepatitis B virus infection. *Hepatology 4*:13.

35. Bertoletti, A., Ferrari, C., Fiaccardori, F., Penna, A., Margolskee, R., Schlicht, H. J., Howler, P., Guilhot, S., Chisari, F. V. (1991). HLA class I-restricted human cy-

totoxic T cells recognize endogenously synthesized hepatitis B virus nucleocapsid antigen. *Proc. Natl. Acad. Sci. 88*:10445–10449.

36. London, W. T., DiFiglia, M., Sutnick, A. I., Blumberg, B. S. (1969). An epidemic of hepatitis in a chronic-hemodialysis unit: Australia antigen and differences in host response. *N. Engl. J. Med. 281*:571–578.

37. Szmuness, W., Prince, A. M., Grady, G. F., et al. (1974). Hepatitis B infection: a point-prevalence study in 15 US hemodialysis centers. *J. Amer. Med. Assoc. 227*:901–906.

38. Tur-Kaspa, R., Burk, R., Shaul, Y., et al. (1986). Hepatitis B virus DNA contains a glucocorticoid-responsive element. *Proc. Natl. Acad. Sci. 83*:1627–1631.

39. Blumberg, B. S., Sutnick, A. I., London, W. T., et al. (1972). Sex distribution of Australia antigen. *Arch. Int. Med. 130*:231.

40. Szmuness, W., Harley, E. J., Ikran, H., et al. (1978). Sociodemographic aspects of the epidemiology of hepatitis B. In: *Viral Hepatitis*, Vyas, G. N., Cohen, S. N. and Schmid, R., (eds). Franklin Institute Press, Philadelphia. p. 297.

41. Liaw, Y. F., Lai, D. I. Chu, C. M., Chen, T. J. (1988). The development of cirrhosis in patients with chronic type B hepatitis: a prospective study. *Hepatology 8*:493–496.

42. Yoakum, G. H., Korba, B. E., Lechner, J. R., et al. (1983). High-frequency transfection and cytopathology of hepatitis B virus core antigen gene in human cells. *Science 222*:385–389.

43. Chisari, F. V. (1991). Analysis of hepadnavirus gene expression, biology, and pathogenesis in the transgenic mouse. *Curr. Top. Microbiol. Immunol. 168*:85–101.

44. Schumacher, H. R., and Gall, E. P. (1974). Arthritis in acute hepatitis and chronic active hepatitis: Pathology of synovial membrane with evidence for the presence of Australia antigen in synovial membranes. *Amer. J. Med. 57*:655.

45. Wands, J. R., Mann, E. A., and Isselbacher, K. J. (1975). The pathogenesis of arthritis associated with acute hepatitis B surface antigen positive hepatitis. Complement activation and characterization of circulating immune complexes. *J. Clin. Invest. 55*:930.

46. Gocke, D. J. (1975). Extrahepatic manifestations of viral hepatitis. *Amer. J. Med. Sci. 270*:49–52.

47. Gocke, J. D. (1975). Immune complex phenomena associated with hepatitis. In: Vyas, G. N., Cohen, S. N., Schmidt. R. (eds). *Viral Hepatitis: A contemporary assessment*. Philadelphia: Franklin Institute Press. p. 27.

48. Robinson, W. S. (1994). Molecular events in the pathogenesis of hepadnavirus-associated hepatocellular carcinoma. *Ann. Rev. Med, 45*:297–323.

49. Beasley, R. P., Lin, C. C., Hwang, L. Y., et al. (1981). Hepatocellular carcinoma and hepatitis B virus: a prospective study of 22,707 men in Taiwan. *Lancet 2*:1129–1133.

50. Obata, H., Hayashi, N. and Motoike, Y. (1980). A prospective study of development of hepatocellular carcinoma from liver cirrhosis with persistent hepatitis B virus infection. *Int. J. Cancer 25*:741.

51. Alward, W. L., McMahon, B. J., Hall, D. B., Heyward, W. L., Francis, D. P., Bender, T. R. (1985). The long-term serologic course of asymptomatic hepatitis B virus carriers and the development of primary hepatocellular carcinoma. *J. Infect. Dis. 151*:604–9.

52. Gerin, J. L. (1990). Experimental WHV infection of woodchucks: an animal model of hepadnavirus-induced liver cancer. *Gastroenterol Jpn 25 Suppl.* 38–42.

53. Korba, B. E., Wells, F. V., Baldwin, B., Cote, P. J., Tennant, B. C., Popper, H., Germ, J. L. (1989). Hepatocellular carcinoma in woodchuck hepatitis virus-infected woodchucks: presence of viral DNA in tumor tissue from chronic carriers and animals serologically recovered from acute infections. *Hepatology 9*:461–70.

54. Marion, P. L., Van Davelaar, M. J., Knight, S. S., Salazar, F. H., Garcia, G., Popper, H. and Robinson W. S. (1983). Hepatocellular carcinoma in ground squirrels persistently infected with ground squirrel hepatitis virus. *Proc. Nat. Acad. Sci. USA 83*:4543–6.

55. Marion, P. L., and Robinson, W. S. Unpublished results.

56. Tiollais, P., Pourcel, C., and Dejean, A. (1985). The hepatitis B virus. *Nature 317*:489–495.

57. Miller, R. H., Lee, S.-C., Liaw, Y.-F., and Robinson, W. S. (1985). Hepatitis B viral DNA in infected human liver and in hepatocellular carcinoma. *J. Inf. Dis. 151*: 1081–92.

58. Dejean, A., Bougueleret, L., Grzeschik, K. H. and Tiollais, P. (1986). Hepatitis B virus DNA integration in a sequence homologous to v-erb A and steroid receptor genes in a hepatocellular carcinoma. *Nature 322*:70–2.

59. Wang, J., Chenivesse, X., Henglein, B., Brechot, C. (1990). Hepatitis B virus integration in a cyclin A gene in a hepatocellular carcinoma. *Nature 343*:555–7.

60. Moroy, T., Marchio, A., Etiemble, J., Trepo, C., Tiollais, P. and Buendia, M. A. (1986). Rearrangement and enhanced expression of c–myc in hepatocellular carcinoma of hepatitis virus infected woodchucks. *Nature 324*:276–9.

61. Hsu, T., Moroy, T., Etiemble, J., Louise, A., Trepo, C., Tiollais, P. and Buendia, M. A. (1988). Activation of c–myc by woodchuck hepatitis virus insertion in hepatocellular carcinoma. *Cell 55*:627–35.

62. Etiemble, J., Moroy, T., Jacquemin, E., Tiollais, P. and Buendia, M. A. (1989). Fused transcripts of c–myc and a new cellular locus, hcr in a primary liver tumor. *Oncogene 4*:51–7.

63. Fourel, G., Trepo, C., Bouqueleret, L, Hemalein, B., Pouzetto, A., Tiollaise, P., and Buendia, M. (1990). Frequent activation of N–myc gene by hepadnavirus insertion in woodchuck liver tumors. *Nature 347*:294–98.

64. Fung, G.-K., Lai, C. L., Todd, D., Ganem, D. and Varmus, H. E. (1984). An amplified domain of cellular DNA containing a subgenomic insert of hepatitis B virus DNA in a human hepatoma. In: *Viral Hepatitis and Liver Disease: The 1984 International Symposium on Viral Hepatitis*, G. Vyas, J. L. Dienstag and J. Hoffnagle (eds). Grune & Stratton, New York, N.Y., p. 633.

65. Fung, G.-K., Lai, C. L., Lok, A., Todd, D. and Varmus, H. E. (1985). Analysis of HBV-associated human hepatocellular carcinoma for oncogene expression and

structure rearrangement. In: *Molecular Biology of Hepatitis B Viruses:* Abstracts of papers presented at the 1985 meeting on molecular biology of hepatitis B viruses, May 2–5, 1985, Varmus, H. (ed.), Cold Spring Harbor, N.Y.: Cold Spring Harbor Laboratory.

66. Transy, C., Fourel, G., Robinson, W. S., Tiollais, P. (1992). Frequent amplification of c–myc in ground squirrel liver tumors associated with past or ongoing infection with a hepadnavirus. *Proc. Natl. Acad. Sci. USA 89*:3874–3878.

67. Hansen, L. J., Tennant, B. C., Seeger, C., Ganem, D. (1993). Differential activation of myc gene family members in hepatic carcinogenesis by closely related hepatitis B viruses. *Mol. Cell Biol. 13*:659–667.

68. Twu, J. S. and Schloemer, R. H. (1987). Transcriptional transactivating functions of hepatitis B virus. *J. Virol. 61*:3448–3453.

69. Twu, J. S., and Robinson, W. S. (1989). Hepatitis B virus x gene can transactivate heterologous viral sequences. *Proc. Natl. Acad. Sci. USA 86*:2046–2050.

70. Seto, E., Yen, T. S., Peterlin, B. M., Ou, J. H. (1988). Trans-activation of the human immunodeficiency virus long terminal repeat by the hepatitis B virus X protein. *Proc. Natl. Acad. Sci. 85*:8286–8290.

71. Siddiqui, A., Gaynor, R., Srinivasan, A., Mapoles, J., and Farr, R. W. (1989). Trans-activation of viral enhancers including long terminal repeat of the human immunodeficiency virus by the hepatitis B virus X protein. *Virology 169*:479–484.

72. Spandau, D. F., and Lee, C. H. (1988). Trans-activation of viral enhancers by the hepatitis B virus X protein. *J. Virol. 62*:427–434.

73. Twu, J. S., Chu, K. and Robinson, W. S. (1989). Hepatitis B virus x-gene activates kB-like enhancer sequences in HIV-1 LTR. *Proc. Natl. Acad. Sci. USA 86*:5168–5172.

74. Zahm, P., Hofschneider, P., Koshy, R. (1988). The HBV X–ORF encodes a trans-activator: a potential factor in viral hepatocarcinogenesis. *Oncogene 3*:169–77.

75. Twu, J. S., Rosen, C. A., Haseltine, W. A. and Robinson, W. S. (1989). Identification of a region within the human immunodeficiency virus (HIV–1) long terminal repeat (LTR) that is essential for transactivation by the hepatitis B virus (HBV) gene X. *J. Virol. 63*:2857–2860.

76. Koike, K., Kobayashi, Yaginama, K., Shirakata, Y. (1987). Structure and function of integrated HBV DNA in: *Hepadnaviruses* ed. W. S. Robinson, K. Koike and H. Will, Alan Liss Inc. New York. P. 267–286.

77. Koike, K., Shirakata, Y., Yaginuma,K., Arii, M., Takada, S., Nakamura, I., Hayashi, Y., Kawada, M., and Kobayashi, M. (1989). Oncogenic potential of hepatitis B virus. *Mol. Biol. Med. 6*:151–160.

78. Twu, J. S., Lai, M.-Y., Chen, D.-H., Robinson, W. S. (1993). Activation of protooncogene C-jun by the x protein of hepatitis B virus. *Virology 192*:346–350.

79. Twu, J. and Robinson, W. S. Unpublished results.

80. Seto, E., Mitchell, J., and Yen, S. B. (1990). Transactivation by the hepatitis B virus x protein depends on AP–2 and other transcription factors. *Nature (London) 344*:72–74.

81. Zhou, D.-X., Taraboulos, A., Ou, J.-H., Benedictyen, T. S. (1990). Activation of class I major histocompatibility complex gene expression by hepatitis B virus. *J. Virol. 64*:4025–4028.

82. Wu, J.-Y., Zhou, Z. Y., Judd, A., Cartwright, C. A. and Robinson, W. S. (1990). The hepatitis B virus-encoded transcriptional transactivator hbx appears to be a novel serine/threonine kinase. *Cell 63*:687–695.

83. Seto, E., Zhou, D.-X., Peterlin, B. M. and Benedictyen, T. S. (1989). Trans-activation by the hepatitis B virus x protein shows cell-type specificity. *Virology 173*:764–766.

84. Hohne, M., Schaefer, S., Seifer, M., Feitelson, M. A., Paul, D., Gerlich, W. H. (1990). Malignant transformation of immortalized transgenic hepatocytes after transfection with hepatitis B virus DNA. *EMBO J. 9*:1137–1145.

85. Kim, C.-M., Koike, K., Saito, I., Miyamura, T., Jay, G. (1991). HBx gene of hepatitis B virus induces liver cancer in transgenic mice. *Nature 351*:317–320.

86. Takada, S., Koike, K. (1990). Trans-activation function of a 3′ truncated X gene-cell fusion product from integrated hepatitis B virus DNA in chronic hepatitis tissues. *Proc. Natl. Acad. Sci. USA 87*:5628–5632.

87. Wollersheim, M., Debelka, U., Hofschneider, P. H. (1988). A transactivating function encoded in the hepatitis B virus X gene is conserved in the integrated state. *Oncogene 3*:545–552.

88. Kekule, A. S., Lauer, U., Meyer, M., Caselmann, W. H., Hofschneider, P. H., Koshy, R. (1990). The preS2/S region of integrated hepatitis B virus DNA encodes a transcriptional transactivator. *Nature 343*:457–461.

89. Caselmann, W. H., Meyer, M., Kekule, A. S., Lauer, U., Hofschneider, P. H., Koshy, R. (1990). A transactivator function is generated by integration of hepatitis B virus preS/S sequences in human hepatocellular carcinoma DNA. *Proc. Natl. Acad. Sci. USA 87*:2970–2974.

90. Trowbridge, R., Fagan, E. A., Davison, F., Eddleston, A. L. W. F., Williams, R., Linskens, M. H. K., and Farzaneh, F. (1988). *Viral Hepatitis and Liver Disease*, ed. Zuckerman, A. J. Liss, New York pp 764–768.

91. Hsu, I. C., Metcalf, R. A., Sun, T., Welsh, J. A., Wang, N. J. and Harris, C. C. (1991). Mutational hotspot in the p53 gene in human hepatocellular carcinomas. *Nature 350*:427–428.

92. Bressac, B., Kew, M., Wands, J., Ozturk, M. (1991). Selective G to T mutations of p53 gene in hepatocellular carcinoma from southern Africa. *Nature 350*:429–431.

93. Buetow, K. H. personal communication.

94. Hosono, S., Lee, C. S., Chou, M. J., Yang, C. S., Shih, C. H. (1991). Molecular analysis of the p53 alleles in primary hepatocellular carcinomas and cell lines. *Onvogene 6*:237–243.

95. Ozturk, M. et al. (1991). p53 mutation in hepatocellular carcinoma after aflatoxin exposure. *Lancet 338*:1356–1359.

96. Rivkina, M. A., Marion, P. L., Robinson, W. S. Unpublished result.

97. Slagle, B. L., Zhou, Y.-Z., and Butel, J. S. (1991). Hepatitis B virus integration event in human chromosome 17p near the p53 gene identifies the region of the

chromosome commonly deleted in virus-positive hepatocellular carcinomas. *Cancer Res. 51*:49–54.

98. Fujimori, M., Tokino, T., Hino, O., Kitagawa, T., Imamura, T., Okamoto, E., Mitsunobu, M., Ishikawa, T., Nakagama, H., Harada, H. (1991). Allelotype study of primary hepatocellular carcinoma. *Cancer Res. 51*:89–93.

99. Bressac, B., Galvin, K. M., Liang, T. J., Isselbacher, K. J., Wands, J. R., Ozturk, M. (1990). Abnormal structure and expression of p53 gene in human hepatocellular carcinoma. *Proc. Natl. Acad. Sci. 87*:1973–1977.

100. Hino, O., Shows, T. B., Rogler, C. E. (1986). Two integrated hepatitis B virus (HBV) DNA molecules were cloned from two primary hepatocellular carcinomas each containing only a single integration. One integration (C3) contained a single linear segment of HBV DNA, and the other integration (C4) contained a large inverted duplication of viral DNA at the site of a chromosome translocation. *Proc. Natl. Acad. Sci. USA 83*:8338–8342.

101. Meyer, M., Wiedorn, K. H., Hofscneider, P. H., Koshy, R., Caselmann, W. H. (1992). A chromosome 17:7 translocation is associated with a hepatitis B virus DNA integration in human hepatocellular carcinoma DNA. *Hepatology 15*:665–671.

102. Gu, J. R. (1988). Molecular aspects of human hepatic carcinogenesis. *Carcinogenesis 9*:697.

103. Yuasa, Y., and Sudo, K. (1987). Transforming genes in human hepatomas detected by a tumorigenicity assay. *Jpn. J. Cancer Res. 78*:1036.

104. Nakagama, H., Ohnishi, S., Imawari, M., Hirai, H., Takaku, F., Sakamoto, H., Terada, M., Nagao, M., and Sugimura, T. (1987). Identification of transforming genes as host in DNA samples from two human hepatocellular carcinomas. *Jpn. J. Cancer Res. 78*:651.

105. Ochiya, T., Fujiyama, A., Fukushige, S., Hatada, I., and Matsubara, K. (1986). Molecular cloning of an oncogene from a human hepatocellular carcinoma. *Proc. Natl. Acad. Sci. USA 83*:4993.

106. Cerutti, P. A. (1988). Response modification creates promotability in multistage carcinogenesis. *Carcinogenesis 9*:519–526.

107. Vesselinovitch, S. D., and Mihailovich, N. (1983). Kinetics of diethylnitrosamine hepatocarcinogenesis in the infant mouse. *Cancer Res. 43*:4253.

108. Scherer, E. (1984). Neoplastic progression in experimental hepatocarcinogenesis. *Biochim. Biophys. Acta 738*:219.

9

Interaction of hepatitis B virus with hepatocytes

Wolfram H. Gerlich and Xuanyong Lu
Institute of Medical Virology
University of Giessen
Frankfurter Strasse 107
D 35392 Giessen, Germany

Introduction

All hepatitis viruses of man are able to persist in cell culture. Hepatitis A virus is not very cytotoxic and can induce persistent infection in cell culture. The fact that it does not persist *in vivo* is due mainly to the very efficient immune elimination. Hepatitis B virus (HBV) is also not cytotoxic at the usual levels of expression, and moreover, it is somehow able to suppress the immune response; it induces a kind of immune tolerance. Cell culture of hepatitis C virus has not yet been achieved, but the observations in patients suggest that, again, its pathogenicity is mostly an immune pathogenicity. In this case, the virus is probably able to persist due to its hypervariable regions in the envelope proteins. Hepatitis Delta virus is also able to replicate and spread from cell to cell without much pathogenicity. If it reaches the serum, it has borrowed the envelope from the hepatitis B virus.

Viremia and Antigenemia

Hepatitis B virus has been named the "Queen of Persistent Viruses" by W. R. Robinson. It is remarkable how constant the pattern of expression is in the persistently infected host. Recently, we studied a group of 45 children who became infected with HBV during cytostatic treatment. Due to that therapy they became completely immune to that virus. They did not show any sign of the disease, neither in the serum with elevated transaminases nor in the liver by conventional histology. However, the degree of viral expression was very similar to highly viremic carriers of hepatitis B virus who were not artificially immune suppressed (Repp et al., 1993).

Virtually all hepatocytes become infected during persistent HBV infection with high viremia. They contain approximately 10 to 100 virus genomes as episomal DNA, and from these episomes, 5 structural proteins are expressed (MacLachlan, 1991, Mason and Seeger, 1991). The core protein HBc, and the viral DNA polymerase assemble together with their messenger RNA as pregenome to the virion core. The virion core is enveloped by the 3 HBs proteins to form the virion, and then these virions are secreted to the blood.

The HBs proteins are produced in excess. They are present not only as components of the virus particles, but also as HBs filaments or as HBs spheres in larger amounts. Typically, a chronically infected carrier, has approximately 100μg HBs spheres, 1 μg HBs filaments, and 0.1 microgram virions per ml serum (Figure 1). This state of viremia and antigenemia is maintained for years and even decades in many persistently infected hosts. This stable state is regulated not only by the gene expression of the virus, but also by the degradation of the virions and the antigens. We believe that most of the antigen actually returns to the liver, where one would expect the receptors for the viral surface proteins. The immune system seems to play a minor role at this stage.

Structure of HBs proteins

This article is mainly devoted to the interaction of hepatic cell membranes with the HBs proteins. Due to secretion, there is much more virus and viral HBsAg in the blood than in the liver. HBsAg particles contain the three HBs proteins: the small, the middle, and the large HBs protein (Figure 1). They form doublets in gel electrophoresis due to partial glycosylation. The small HBs protein is the major component of the virus itself, the filamentous form and the spherical form of HBsAg. The middle HBs pro-

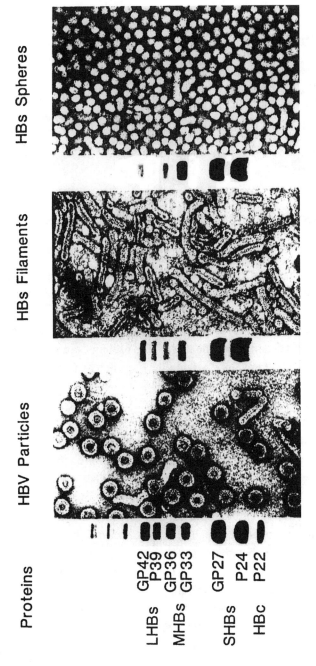

Figure 1 HBV-associated particles and proteins purified from the plasma of a low-symptomatic chronic HBV carrier. 200 ml plasma yielded approximately 500 µl of purified virions, 11 ml HBs filaments and 5 ml of HBs spheres. Ten µl of the preparation were applied to electron microscopy grids or to SDS gels either undiluted or 1:10 for HBs spheres. Grids were stained with uranylacetate, gels with silver.

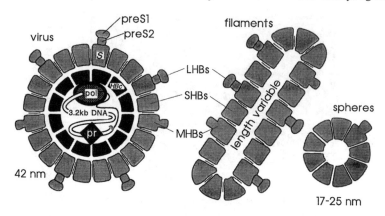

Figure 2 Model of the HBV virions, HBs filaments and HBs spheres.

tein is a minor component in all three particle forms, whereas the large
HBs protein is almost absent in the 20 nm–particles, which are abundant
(Heermann et al., 1984; Heermann and Gerlich, 1991).

Figure 2 shows a model of the virus and the HBs particles. The small
HBs protein, and the S domain of the larger HBs proteins, are very hydrophobic and form a solid envelope around the capsid. The middle protein
contains a preS2 domain, and the larger protein contains a preS1 and
preS2 domain. Both of these domains are very hydrophilic and accessible
at the surface of the virus.

The spatial structure of the small HBs proteins, and of the S domains of
the larger HBs protein, are not exactly known, but the following data suggest the model drawn in Figure 3. Circular dichroism shows that approximately 60% of the polypeptide is in an alphahelical configuration. All
algorithms for secondary structure predictions suggest that these alphahelices are in highly hydrophobic sequence regions. *In vitro* processing (Ganem, 1991) has shown that the first aminoterminal alphahelix would
insert into the membrane of the ER with the aminoterminus facing the lumen. The second alphahelix inserts again into the membrane, but now in
the opposite orientation. Both of these alphahelices have translocation
functions. Helix I transports the upstream, helix II the downstream protein sequences to the lumen of the ER. The hypothetical alphahelices III

and IV are, according to computer predictions, multimerizing, transmembranous helices (Berting et al., 1995). If these predictions are valid the model of Figure 3 is a logical consequence. A similar model has also been deduced by Stirk et al. (1992).

The aminoterminal hydrophilic region faces toward the internal side of the particles, and the central hydrophilic region forms the HBs epitopes, which are found on the surface of the virus and the HBs particles.

Attachment of HBV

According to our knowledge the classical HBs Ag does not participate in the interactions of the virus or the HBs particles with liver cells; at least, we and most other investigators could not identify any attachment of this site with hepatic cells. There is probably attachment of the preS2 domain in the middle HBs protein to hepatocytes (Pontisso et al., 1989). The group of Barnaba has shown that the preS2 region may probably bind to the transferrin receptor of T cells, and then it is taken up by these cells (Franco et al., 1992).

It is also known that the central part of the preS2 domain binds a kind of modified human serum albumin (Krone et al., 1990), and this modified human serum albumin has an affinity for liver cells. Moreover, my coworker Lu Xuanyong could show that the tri-antennary glycoside at the amino end of preS2 has a hepatocyte-specific composition of monosaccharides, and that it binds to human hepatoma cells (unpublished). The preS2 glycan has an unusual composition, and we believe that the arrangement of the monosaccharides in the tri-antennary glycan binds to a novel lectin that we have not yet identified. This lectin is not present in normal human liver, but it is present in significant amounts in HepG2 cells. We speculate that this lectin may be related to the growth or differentiation status of the cell.

The best characterized attachment site of hepatitis B virus resides in the large HBs protein in the sequence 21 to 47 in the preS1 domain. This site attaches to human hepatoma cells and to various leukocytic cell lines, as was shown first by Neurath et al. (1986). In order to study whether this site also attaches to natural human liver, my collaborators in Padova, repeated that experiment (Pontisso et al., 1989). They isolated, from surgi-

Small HBs Protein

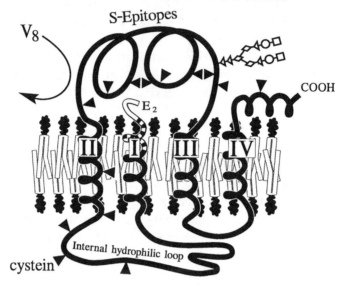

Middle HBs Protein

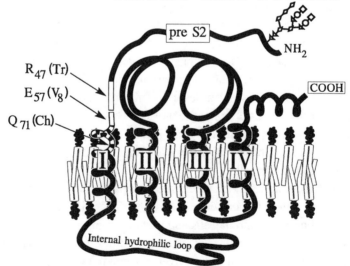

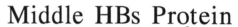

Large HBs Protein (Virion)

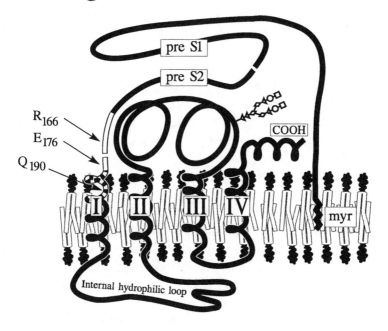

Figure 3 Topological model of the three co-terminal HBs proteins and the viral lipid membrane. The Roman numerals delineate the four postulated transmembraneous alphahelices. The cleavage sites of Va protease, trypsin (tr) and chymotrypsin (ch) are shown. The section of the polypeptide shown in white is the proteolysis sensitive site. The hatched part is the hypothetical fusion site.

cally obtained liver specimens, liver plasma membranes. HBs filaments and virions, which contain much of the preS1 domain, bound quite well to such membranes. This binding could be specifically inhibited by a monoclonal antibody to the sequence 31 to 34 of the preS1 domain, whereas other monoclonal antibodies against other sequence of HBs proteins were not able to inhibit that attachment.

This attachment site is probably involved in the infection process because antibodies against that region are able to neutralize infectivity of hepatitis B virus for chimpanzees (Neurath & Thanavala, 1990). One potential model for how hepatitis B virus could escape immune surveillance would be that this important attachment site would be hypervariable. To study this postulate we analyzed the variability in 24 HBV isolates from northern Germany. In the literature up to 30% variability were reported in the preS1 attachment region. We wanted to see how this seemingly highly variable sequence is conserved during infection chains. An example of an infection chain was a surgeon who infected six of his patients while operating. Other examples were transmissions between couples, between mother and child, and a small outbreak of hepatitis B in a dialysis ward. Twenty-five samples of genotype A were sequenced, and surprisingly little variation was found. In 18 of the 25 sera the sequences were completely identical with a previously published sequence. In three sera we found one exchange, in two sera another exchange, and in another couple we found two exchanges (Uy et al., 1992). We conclude from this data that variability cannot be the reason for persistence of hepatitis B virus in the presence of a functioning immune system. The sequence was completely identical within the different infection groups, and three sera from the surgeon collected in a time period of four years were also completely identical.

Table 1 summarizes reports on potential or real attachment sites of HBV to various cell membranes. PreS1 binds to a cell-bound interleukin 6 (IL6), which is present on various types of white blood cells, and also on hepatic cells (Neurath et al., 1992). Pontisso et al. (1992) suggested that this attachment competes with IgA; the preS1 receptor would then be a novel IgA receptor. It is not clear if this receptor is identical with the IL–6-related structure. The glycan of preS2 may also be an attachment site to liver cells. Guido Gerken from Mainz has recently suggested that the preS domain might bind to the asialoglycoprotein receptor from liver cells (Treichel et al., 1994), but our own data suggest that an unknown novel glycan could also be a receptor. The preS1 domain may also interact with modified serum albumin or the transferrin receptor. Finally there are two groups who suggest that the S domain may contribute to attachment (Hertogs et al., 1994, Mehdi et al., 1994).

Table 9.1. *Interactions of HBV surface proteins with host proteins*

Domain	Host protein	Reference
preS1 (21–47)	Hepatocyte membrane protein HBV-BF	2
preS1 (21–47)	cell bound IL6	18
preS1 (23–47)	(modified ?) IgA	19
preS	asialoglycoprotein receptor	25
preS2 glycoside	unknown lectin of HepG2 cells	
preS2 (133–145)	transferrin receptor	3
preS2 (130–150)	modified human serum albumin	19
S	(modified ?) apolipoprotein H	15
S	hepatocyte endonexin II	7

Protease-induced infectivity

There is one great weakness of all published studies on attachment: the systems are not connected with proven infectivity of the virus. For instance, human hepatoma cells HepG2 cells are known to contain two efficient attachment sites: the preS1 site, and the preS2 glycan. Nevertheless they cannot be efficiently infected. In contrast, liver membranes, for instance, do not contain the receptor for the preS2 glycan; instead, they contain the receptor for the preS2-bound polymerized human serum albumin. *In vivo*, the natural liver cell is susceptible and can be readily infected. One may, therefore, speculate that the preS2-albumin complex is important for infectivity *in vivo*.

Recently, Budkowska et al. (1993) have observed a HBV-binding factor which is present on the surface of hepatocytes obtained from liver biopsies but not on Hep2 cells. This not-yet-identified protein may be a HBV receptor.

Something is obviously lacking in the cell culture systems to which HBV attaches. An essential factor which could be missing could be a suitable protease. Most envelope viruses need a hydrophobic fusion sequence which allows the entry of the nucleocapsid into the cell after activation by proteolytic cleavage. In the genome of hepatitis B virus, we find a protease hypersensitive region at the transition from the preS2 domain to the S domain. This region can be cleaved *in vitro* easily by various proteases, including trypsin, V8-protease, or chymotrypsin. It is interesting to note that this site is next to a hydrophobic region which is similar to known fusion sequences of other enveloped viruses. We tested that hypothesis in the following way: we purified and enriched hepatitis B virus from virus carrier plasma by sucrose gradient centrifugation, treated the purified viruses with V8-protease, chymotrypsin, or nothing, and then the proteases were removed by a second centrifugation. This pretreated virus was given to HepG2 cells, and the intracellular appearance of HBsAg was followed. With untreated virus, or chymotrypsin-treated virus, we did not find intracellular HBsAg, whereas after treatment with V8 protease, we found an increase of intracellular HBsAg. After 6 days the HBsAg decreased again, but after 20 days we found a second peak, and this suggests that an infection has occurred. The appearance of newly synthesized HBV DNA was also followed. The DNA was detected by amplification in PCR. We were able to detect approximately 1 to 10 virions per cell. It was possible to infect HepG2 cells by a treatment of the virus with V8 protease, whereas untreated virus or chymotrypsin-treated virus did not generate intracellular HBV DNA. The signal strengths correlated well with the amount of virus which is found in a transfected HepG2 cell (HepG22.15). That the HBV DNA was newly formed is shown by the kinetics of the HBV DNA production within the cell. After 2 days and 5 days no intracellular HBV genomes were detected at the level of sensitivity which was applied. However, after 6 days, a very strong signal appeared.

The newly formed virus is also secreted. The supernatant of the infected cells again generated a strong PCR signal after days 5 and 6, which decreased there-after; such a signal was not found with untreated virus or with chymotrypsin-treated virus. For the assay of secreted HBV, the cell supernatant was precipitated with a monoclonal antibody against the preS2 region, and the immune precipitate was analyzed by PCR. Please consider that the V8 protease treatment removed the preS2 domain, and the ability to precipitate that virus with a preS2 antibody showed that this was really newly formed virus (Lu et al., 1996).

Characteristics of the potential fusion site

How can one explain the effect of the V8 protease? This protease cleaves only at the transition between the preS2 domain and the S domain exactly where the proteolysis-sensitive and the hydrophobic region are. We would postulate that cleavage at this region induces the infectivity of V8 protease-treated HBV for HepG2 cells. There is, however, one problem in that model. The small HBs protein has the fusion sequence in exactly the same structure as it is generated by V8 protease from middle or large HBs protein.

Thus, the question was whether the preS2 domain is necessary at all for the protease-induced infectivity. The treatment with V8 protease not only induced infectivity of hepatitis B virus for HepG2 cells, but it also induces nonspecific binding of the surface proteins to all kind of cell membranes. This binding is acid resistant and irreversible. Now we used recombinant HBsAg particles, either with or without the middle HBs protein and studied the protease-induced binding to cell membranes. Binding occurred only if the middle HBs-protein was present, and it was abolished by treatment with chymotrypsin. Particles which contained only the small HBs proteins did not irreversibly bind.

How can we explain this finding? We postulate that the aminoterminus of the S domain, which we presume to be a fusion sequence, is hidden in the small HBs protein, and that it is accessible in the middle HBs protein after proteolysis. To show this we stained the HBs protein at the amino terminus covalently with a chemical named DABITC and digested the stained HBs particles with nothing, V8 protease, or with V8 protease after lysis by SDS. The rationale was that the glutamic acid next to the amino terminus of the S domain would only be cleaved by the V8 protease, if it was accessible. A densitometric scan of the DABITC-labeled HBs proteins showed the 24 kD and 27 kD small HBs protein and 33 kD middle HBs protein. After treatment of the particles with V8 protease the stain was not removed, whereas the stain from the middle HBs was removed because this site is accessible for V8 protease. We could only remove the DABITC stain from the small HBs protein when the particles were first lysed with SDS.

Based on this result, we believe that the amino terminus is somehow
hidden within the small molecule and is not accessible to the surface of
the HBs particles or virions. In contrast, in the middle and large HBs proteins, the presence of the preS domains would force the aminoterminal S
domain to a more exposed position, and then this position would be accessible to protease. It is very important for the viral life cycle that this
region is not prematurely exposed, as with other fusion sequences, because in the activated configuration, the HBsAg and HBV would bind to
all kinds of cells, for instance mouse fibroblasts or HeLa cells as we have
shown. It is interesting to note that this type of unspecific cell membrane
binding of HBsAg is pH dependent. It has its optimum at pH 5.5 and this
suggests that the binding may actually occur in the endosome (Lu and
Gerlich, 1996).

Entry of HBV into hepatocytes

These data lead to a model of how hepatitis B virus enters hepatocytes.
The first attachment may be between the preS1 domain (sequence 21 to
47) and its not-yet-identified receptor. This attachment is not hepatocyte
specific, it occurs also with leukocytes and with the hepatoma cell line
HepG2 which cannot be infected. One may presume that there is no endocytosis, and that the preS1 receptor is incomplete. Probably another, closer attachment is necessary for which several candidate receptors exist.
This may be the preS2 glycoside which could bind, for instance, with the
asialoglycoprotein receptor. It may be the transferrin receptor, or binding
and endocytosis may be indirect by a modified human serum albumin,
which then would be processed within the hepatocyte. Once endocytosis
has occurred, the lower pH of the late endosome would allow for proteolysis at the transition with the preS2 domain and the S domain. This would
liberate the fusion sequence and the nucleoprotein of HBV could be released to the cytosol. We believe that this model has some reality because
in our artificial system we could induce viral entry from outside with a
protease-treated HBV at pH 5.5.

Oncogenicity of HBV

Virtually all DNA viruses of mammals encode proteins which exert a positive effect on cellular growth regulation, e.g. the E6, E7 proteins of papillomaviruses, the E1A and E1B proteins of adenoviruses or the tumor antigen of polyomaviruses. Recently we have obtained evidence that the X protein of hepatitis B virus is a viral oncogene. Previously we have shown that an immortalized mouse hepatocyte line (FMH 202) which contains an SV40 TAg antigen is not tumorigenic but can be converted to tumorigenicity by transfection with HBV DNA. Such HBV expressing cell clones grew in soft agar and in nude mice very well, whereas the original clone could not (Höhne et al., 1990).

We repeated this type of experiment with a cloned X gene of the HBV genome, under the control of its own enhancer and promoter. For control, we used an X gene construct with a stop codon instead of codon 23. We saw that the stably transfected clones with the mutated X gene could not grow in soft agar, whereas the clones which expressed a reasonable amount of X mRNA grew moderately well in soft agar and, after a while, these clones developed tumors in nude mice. This, in our opinion, is proof that X protein of HBV is really a viral tumor protein (Seifer et al., 1991, Seifer and Gerlich, 1992). What does X protein do in this system? Among other effects we found that it alters tumor suppressor protein p53 in the nucleus. FMH 202 cells containing mutated X gene show the normal intracellular distribution of p53 in a nuclear position. In the X expressing cells, the p53 is no longer detectable in the nucleus. This is not a defect in the nuclear transport because the SV40T antigen, which also contains cells, is hyper-phosphorylated and conformationally altered. We were, however, not able to detect a direct interaction between the X protein and p53 (Schaefer et al., unpublished). X protein has been characterized as a weak nonspecific transcriptional activator, which can induce production of diacylglycerol and activation of protein kinase C (Kekulé et al., 1993). The mode of how X protein alters p53 remains, however, unclear at present.

Acknowledgement

The work from our group was supported by DFG grants to W.H.G. (SFB 249/A12 and SFB 272/C4).

References

1. Berting, A., J. Hahnen, M. Kröger, and W. H. Gerlich. (1995). Computer-aided studies on the topology of small hepatitis B surface protein. *Intervirology 38*:8–15.

2. Budkowska, A., C. Quan, F. Groh, P. Bedessa, P. Dubreuil, J. P. Bouvet, and J. Pillot. (1993). Hepatitis B virus (HBV) binding factor in human serum: candidate for a soluble form of hepatocyte HBV receptor. *J. Virol. 67*:4316–4322.

3. Franco, A., M. Paroli, U. Testa, R. Benvenuto, C. Peschle, F. Balsano, and V. Barnaba. (1992). Transferrin receptor mediates uptake and presentation of hepatitis B envelope antigen by T lymphocytes. *J. Exp. Med. 175*:1195–1205.

4. Ganem, D. (1991). *Assembly of hepadnaviral virions and subviral particles*. In: Mason W. S., and C. Seeger eds. Hepadnaviruses–Molecular Biology and Pathogenesis. Curr. Top. Microbiol. Immunol. Vol. 168: 61–84, Springer Verlag, Berlin.

5. Heermann, K. -H., and W. H. Gerlich. (1991). *Surface proteins of hepatitis B viruses*. In: Mac Lachlan, A., ed. Molecular Biology of Hepatitis B Viruses, Boca Raton: CRC.

6. Heermann, K.-H., U. Goldmann, W. Schwartz, T. Seyffarth, H. Baumgarten, and W. H. Gerlich. (1984). Large surface proteins of hepatitis B virus containing the pre-S sequence. *J. Virol. 52:* 396–402.

7. Hertogs, K., E. Depla, T. Crabbe, W. De Bruin, W. Leenders, M. Moshage, and S. H. Yap. (1994). Spontaneous development of anti-hepatitis B virus envelope (anti-idiotypic) antibodies in animals immunized with human liver endonexin II immunoglobulin G: Evidence for a receptor–ligand-like relationship between small hepatitis B virus surface antigen and endonexin II. *J. Virol. 68*:1516–1521.

8. Höhne, M., S. Schaefer, M. Seifer, M. A. Feitelson, D. Paul, and W. H. Gerlich. (1990). Malignant transformation of immortalized transgenic hepatocytes after transfection with hepatitis B virus DNA. *EMBO J. 9*:1137–1145.

9. Kekulé, A. S., H. Lauer, L. Weiss, B. Luber, and P. H. Hofschneider. (1993). Hepatitis B virus transactivation HBx uses a tumour promoter signalling pathway. *Nature 361*:742–745.

10. Krone, B., A. Lenz, K.-H. Heermann, M. Seifer, X. Lu, and W. H. Gerlich. (1990). Interaction between hepatitis B surface proteins and monomeric human serum albumin. *Hepatology 11*:1050–1056.

11. Lu, X. and W. H. Gerlich. (1996). Proteolysis-induced binding of a fusion peptide-like structure in hepatitis B surface antigen to cellular membranes, submitted.

12. Lu, X., T. Block and W. H. Gerlich. (1996). Protease-induced infectivity of hepatitis B virus for a human hepatoblastoma cell. *J. Virol 70*:2277–2285.

13. Mason, W. S., and C. Seeger, eds. (1991). Hepadnaviruses–Molecular Biology and Pathogenesis. *Curr. Top. Microbiol. Immunol. 168*:61–84, Springer Verlag, Berlin.

14. MacLachlan, A., ed. (1991). Molecular Biology of Hepatitis B Viruses, CRC Press, Boca Raton.

15. Mehdi, H., M. J. Kaplan, F. Y. Anlar, X. Yang, R. Bayer, K. Sutherland and M. E. Peeples. (1994). Hepatitis B virus surface antigen binds to apolipoprotein H. *J. Virol. 68*:2415–2424.

16. Neurath A. R., S. B. H. Kent, N. Strick, K. Parker. (1986). Identification and chemical synthesis of a host cell receptor binding site on hepatitis B virus. *Cell* 46:429–436.
17. Neurath, A. R., and Y. Thanavala. (1990). *Hepadnaviruses*. In: M. H. V. van Regenmortel and A. R. Neurath, eds. Immunochemistry of viruses II. Elsevier, Amsterdam, 403–458.
18 Neurath, A. R., N. Strick, and Y. Y. Li. (1992). Cells transfected with human interleukin 6 cDNA acquire binding sites for the hepatitis B virus envelope protein. *J. Exp. Med. 176*:1561–1569.
19. Pontisso, P., M. G. Ruvoletto, W. H. Gerlich, K.-H. Heermann, R. Bordine, and A. Alberti. (1989). Identification of an attachment site for human liver plasma membranes on hepatitis B virus particles. *Virology 173*: 522–530.
20. Pontisso, P., M. G. Ruvoletto, C. Tiribelli, W. H. Gerlich, A. Ruol, and A. Alberti. (1992). The preS1 domain of hepatitis B virus and IgA cross-react in their binding to hepatocyte surface. *J. Gen. Virol. 73*: 2041–2045.
21. Repp, R., B. V. Hörsten, A. Csecke, J. Kreuder, A. Borkhardt, W. R. Willems, F. Lampert, and W. H. Gerlich. (1993). Clinical and immunological aspects of hepatitis B virus infection in children receiving multidrug cancer chemotherapy. *Arch. Virol. Suppl. 8*:103–111.
22. Seifer M., M. Höhne, S. Schaefer and W. H. Gerlich. (1991). In vitro–tumorigenicity of hepatitis B virus DNA and HBx protein. *J. Hepatol. 13, Suppl. 4*:61–65.
23. Seifer M. and W. H. Gerlich. (1992). Increased growth of permanent mouse fibroblasts in soft agar after transfection with hepatitis B virus DNA. *Arch. Virol. 126*:119–128.
24. Stirk, H. J., J. M. Thornton, and C. R. Howard. (1992). A topological model for hepatitis B surface antigen. *Intervirology 33*:148–158.
25. Treichel, U., K. -H. Meyer zum Büschenfelde, R. I. Stockert, T. Poralla and G. Gerken. (1994). The asialyglycoprotein receptor mediates hepatic uptake of natural hepatitis B virus derived from viremic carriers. *J. Gen. Virol. 75*:3021–3029.
26. Uy, A., G. Wunderlich, D. B. Olsen, K.-H. Heermann, W. H. Gerlich, and R. Thomssen. (1992). Genomic variability in the preS1 region and determination of transmission routes of hepatitis B virus. *J. Gen. Virol. 73*:3005–3009.

10

Viral hemorrhagic fevers: persistent problems, persistent in reservoirs

C. J. Peters
Special Pathogens Branch
Division of Viral and Rickettsial Diseases
National Center for Infectious Diseases
Centers for Disease Control and Prevention
Atlanta, Georgia 30333, USA

James W. LeDuc
Division of Communicable Diseases
World Health Organization
Geneva, Switzerland

For most of the viruses discussed in this book, man is the reservoir, and the virus is either maintained by latency, reactivation, or perhaps by continuous transmission from man to man. For a large number of viruses that infect humans and cause disease, however, inter-human spread is not an important feature of maintenance. While this distinction may seem anthropocentric, it provides an instructive epidemiologic perspective. This discussion will show some of the ways by which these viruses maintain themselves and point out some of the unappreciated regularities in their strategies for survival.

We will concentrate on the viruses that cause hemorrhagic fever. Machupo virus, shown on the front of this volume, is an example. It is a

Table 10.1. *Similarities and differences of hemorrhagic fever viruses*

Similarities	Differences
Vascular syndrome	Replication strategies differ
Dysregulation	Negative sense
Increased permeability	Positive sense
Damage	Ambisense
Small RNA viruses, ca $1–2\times10^6$	Particle formation and morphology
Dalton genome	Cytopathic effects in mammalian cells may be nil or severe
Lipid envelope	
Aerosol infectivity	Antiviral effects of interferon may be minimal or potent
Persist in nature	Nature of human immune response

member of the family *Arenaviridae* and is the cause of a serious, life-threatening disease called Bolivian hemorrhagic fever. This disease and other viral hemorrhagic fevers represent a disease syndrome. They are marked by abnormalities of the vascular system, which allow them to be classed together by their clinical manifestations, but they are etiologically diverse and there are several different pathogenetic mechanisms (Peters, 1996). The causative agents are small RNA viruses with a lipid envelope. They are usually aerosol infectious, for reasons that are not clear (Table 1). They comprise at least four different virus families, and in at least one of those families, there are three different genera responsible for these diseases (Table 2). These viruses are public health problems and will re-main so for the foreseeable future as a result of the persistence mecha-nisms that have evolved to assure their continued natural maintenance in the face of ecologic adversity. These mechanisms are not well understood at the viral or host genetic level but exhibit regularities in biologic strate-gies. These regularities will be used as a basis for speculation concerning the unknown natural history of filoviruses.

Table 10.2.   *The major viral hemorrhagic fevers*

TAXON	VIRUS	DISEASE
ARENAVIRIDAE		
New World	Machupo	Bolivian hemorrhagic fever
	Junin	Argentine hemorrhagic fever
	Guanarito	Venezuelan hemorrhagic fever
	Sabia	Brazilian hemorrhagic fever
Old World	Lassa	Lassa fever
BUNYAVIRIDAE		
Phlebovirus	Rift Valley fever	Rift Valley fever
Nairovirus	Crimean Congo hemorrhagic fever	Crimean Congo hemorrhagic fever
Hantavirus	Hantaan	Hemorrhagic fever with renal syndrome
	Seoul	
	Puumala	
	Sin Nombre	Hantavirus pulmonary syndrome
	Black Creek Canal	
FILOVIRIDAE	Marburg	Marburg hemorrhagic fever
	Ebola	Ebola hemorrhagic fever
FLAVIVIRIDAE	Yellow fever	Yellow fever
	Dengue viruses (1–4)	Dengue hemorrhagic fever

Less common species of the genus *Hantavirus* causing both syndromes are omitted. The tick-borne flavivirus diseases Omsk hemorrhagic fever and Kyasanur forest disease and their viruses are also not included.

Each of these viruses has the capability to persist in at least one of the non-human hosts involved in their transmission cycle (Table 3). In the case of the arenaviruses and the hantaviruses, the rodent host will be chronically infected. With the arthropod-borne viruses, the mosquito or tick vector is chronically infected, and the mammalian host is acutely in-

Table 10.3.   *Hemorrhagic fever viruses: properties and reservoirs*

TAXON	RESERVOIR*	CYTOPATHIC EFFECT+	INTERFERON^
Arenavirus	Rodent	Slight	Slight
Phlebovirus	Mosquito	None	Marked
Nairovirus	Tick	None	Marked
Hantavirus	Rodent	Slight	Marked
Filovirus	Unknown	Unknown	Slight
Flavivirus	Mosquito	None	Marked

*Reservoir host that develops persistent infection
+CPE in cells cultured from reservoir host
^Sensitivity to antiviral effects of mammalian alpha interferon

fected. All these hosts are relatively short-lived, unlike humans who migrate long distances and live for a long time with the possibilities of recrudescence or virus shedding. Most rodents and mosquitoes in the wild live for less than one year, so that intergenerational transmission becomes a very important issue in the natural persistence of these viruses. Thus, it is not surprising that there is usually a linkage mechanism that assures transmission to the next generation of animal host. The persistence strategies of hemorrhagic fever viruses are summarized in Table 4.

Rift Valley fever virus

As an example, Rift Valley fever (RVF) virus is a phlebovirus that has been found in most areas of sub-Saharan Africa. The virus was discovered as an epizootic disease in domestic animals. Tremendous epizootics rapidly spread through herds of sheep and cattle, resulting in nearly 100% abortion among pregnant animals, considerable morbidity and mortality among young and adult animals, and secondary transmission to humans. The epidemics were recognized in areas of Africa in which imported sheep and cattle were kept in large numbers and they occurred during times of exceptionally heavy rainfall that resulted in dense mosquito populations. The epidemiology in this situation was quickly described: in-

Table 10.4. *Persistence strategies of hemorrhagic fever viruses*

FAMILY/GENUS	HORIZONTAL	INTERGENERATIONAL
Arenaviridae	***Rodent–Rodent***	Congenital
Bunyaviridae		
Phlebovirus	***Mosquito*–Mammal**	Transovarial
Nairovirus	***Tick*–Mammal**	Transtadial; some transovarial
Hantavirus	***Rodent–Rodent***	Horizontal
Filoviridae	Unknown	Unknown
Flaviviridae	***Mosquito*–Mammal**	Occasional transovarial

Bold italics indicate persistent infection in that host.

fected sheep or cattle develop very high virus titers in blood; uninfected mosquitoes take a bloodmeal from viremic hosts and become infected; and after an extrinsic incubation period, they may pass the infection along to susceptible vertebrate hosts at subsequent feeding. These mosquitoes are not just mechanical carriers but undergo infection, with the equivalent of viremic dissemination to organs such as salivary glands. This results in their ability to transmit the virus at bloodfeeding throughout the duration of their lives (Faran et al., 1986; Faran et al., 1988; Peters and Linthicum, 1994).

This cycle was seen repeatedly, but the questions arose: How did the virus persist between epidemics? What was its endemic disease activity? What form did RVF take before large sheep and cattle ranches were introduced to Africa? To address these questions, field studies were conducted in endemic areas of Africa. The Central African Republic offered interesting opportunities to explore these questions; it has not adopted cattle or sheepherding as a major industry as have many of the other countries where major rainy–season epidemics have been described. Nevertheless, marked climatic contrasts exist. The southern regions are moist and wet, and the country becomes progressively drier until the northeast, where it is seasonally quite arid. A serosurvey of residents of the rain forest areas found that only about 2.5% had antibodies to RVF virus. Progressing north into drier areas, there was an antibody prevalence of 13.5% in the moist savannahs, 11% in the dry savannah, and 15% antibody prevalence in the driest steppe areas of the northeast. These antibodies represent endemic infection from whatever the reservoir or persistence mechanism that the virus uses in this habitat. There was no correlation with the overall rainfall. Rather the areas with the highest antibody prevalence rates were characterized by generally arid conditions, but with seasonal rainfall leading to flooding and vigorous growth of grasses for part of the year.

Examination of the literature produced no evidence for the possibility that wild vertebrates were involved in the natural persistence of RVF virus. No evidence was found for chronic infection in any of the animals that had been tested in a laboratory setting, and birds and reptiles did not even become infected or viremic (reviewed in Peters and LeDuc, 1991; Peters and Anderson, 1981). Resistant mammalian hosts may experience a limited infection, with localized cells perhaps infected and detectable histologically, but without disseminated infection or significant viremia. In a susceptible host, the infection spreads with high viremia, and necrosis occurs in infected tissues. There is no evidence for latency in non-arthropods, beyond the ability to cocultivate the virus at a maximum of a few weeks post infection.

With regard to the invertebrate host, RVF virus has been isolated from many different genera of mosquitoes captured in nature. The diversity of species found infected does not indicate that all are significantly involved in the maintenance of the virus, but rather probably reflects the extremely high titers of virus circulating during acute infection of the epizootic vertebrate hosts, sheep, and cattle (Turell and Bailey, 1987). If sufficient virus is ingested by a mosquito during bloodfeeding, there is relatively little mosquito species specificity to infection. Once infected, the invertebrate host experiences a silent, largely non-cytopathic infection, which does not appear to overtly affect its longevity or reproductive potential. In addition to salivary glands and other tissues, fat tissues, which serve a function similar to the liver in vertebrates, and neuronal tissues are infected. Interestingly, these tissues are also common target organs in mammals infected with RVF virus (Faran et al., 1986; Faran et al., 1988).

Examination of both the mammals and the mosquitoes, either alone or in combination, failed to reveal an epidemiologic linkage that could explain the persistence of the virus in nature. Even with the persistent infection of the mosquito after bloodfeeding, the seasonally very dry habitat found in many disease–endemic areas seemed very unlikely to support continued virus transmission between vertebrates and vector mosquitoes for the full year. Thus, a mechanism for virus persistence during this interepidemic/epizootic period was still required to fully explain the basis of virus endemicity. Two clues were extremely helpful in unravelling this story. Dr. Robert Swanepoel, a virologist then working in Zimbabwe, examined sites of epizootic transmission of RVF in cattle during 1978 and 1979 (Swanepoel, 1981). The time course of epizootic RVF was important; they did not start in one place and spread elsewhere, as might be expected for an introduction of virus, as observed in many influenza outbreaks. Instead, disease was found in cattle in many areas of the country at more or less the same time, corresponding to the establishment of the rainy season. This was suggestive of a common, widespread mechanism of virus persistence during the dry season. Parenthetically, RVF virus is monotypic; there is no evidence of immune selection on the virus, even if strains collected from all over Africa are examined (Battles and Dalrymple, 1988).

Next, the ecologic features of sites where outbreaks had started were examined. An association was noted between the presence of soil depressions, frequently called "vleies" or "dambos," which accumulate water during the rains, and the sites where epizootic transmission was first noted. Dambos occur not only in Zimbabwe, but also throughout much of sub-Saharan Africa and are central to the life cycle of floodwater mosquitoes of the genus *Aedes*. After bloodfeeding, these mosquitoes deposit their eggs around the margin of dambos. The eggs are drought resistant and lie dormant until subsequent rains. Rainfall must be substantial to trigger hatching; actual flooding must occur; then, the next generation of mosquitoes develops through the larval and pupal stages and emerges as adult mosquitoes about one week after hatching (Davies et al., 1985).

Larval mosquitoes were collected from naturally flooded dambos in RVF enzootic areas and transported to a laboratory, where they were reared to the adult stage, and then examined for the presence of RVF virus. A total of 14 isolations were made from mosquitoes reared from lar-vae. Since they had no opportunity to obtain a bloodmeal, they had no chance of acquiring the virus from a vertebrate host. Thus, they must have already been infected at the time of hatching. Additionally, some of those found infected were males, which do not feed on blood (Linthicum et al., 1985). Together, these observations strongly supported the pre-sumption of transovarial transmission. To confirm this suspicion, the dambos were artificially flooded the following year, and once again in-fected mosquitoes with no possibility of bloodfeeding were recovered. The species that appears to be most important in maintenance of RVF vi-rus is *Ae. macintoshi* formerly known as *Ae. lineatopennis,* whereas mos-quitoes of other species and genera, such as *Culex,* do not appear to contribute to the cycle. Unfortunately, *Ae. macintoshi* has proven ex-tremely difficult to colonize in the laboratory, so the entire cycle has not been demonstrated under controlled conditions. Confirmation is still re-quired. Nonetheless, this pattern is ecologically virtually identical to that of other *Aedes*-borne viruses of the family *Bunyaviridae* that have been investigated in greater detail (LeDuc, 1979; Peters and LeDuc, 1991).

The persistence mechanism in nature therefore involves a persistently infected mosquito passing the infection to the eggs, which are deposited at the margin of a dambo. The eggs, also persistently infected, remain dormant for months or perhaps even years, until the dambo is flooded, at which time they hatch and the next generation of mosquitoes develops and emerges as adults, already infected through transstadial transmission of the virus. When these newly emerged adults take a bloodmeal, they ini-tiate a non-persistent infection in susceptible vertebrates. The transiently viremic host is then fed upon by uninfected mosquitoes, resulting in spreading horizontal infection, more persistently infected adult mosqui-toes, and oviposition of infected mosquito eggs to assure perpetuation of the virus. The requirement for dessication and then immersion in water for initiation of the developmental program of these "flood-water" *Aedes* mosquitoes fits in well with the ecology of places such as the seasonally arid northeastern Central African Republic. Epizootics in areas such as Kenya rely on the flooding of dambos to initiate virus transmission and exceptionally high rainfall to provide the swarms of mosquitoes (not usually the reservoir *Aedes)* for maintenance of high rates of virus transmission among livestock.

Significant interventions can now be proposed on the basis of natural maintenance. Prediction of epidemics and detection of dambos may be possible using satellite based remote sensing (Linthicum et al, 1991). Water management and controlled release of larvicides (e.g., Dursban) may reduce the chance for initiation of RVF virus transmission, and this approach has proved feasible under experimental conditions (Logan et al, 1990). Also, timed vaccination of domestic animals can be performed to protect vulnerable species when they are most likely to be fed upon by infected mosquitoes. However, none of these approaches would be expected to eradicate the virus because of the persistence of viral genome in hardy mosquito eggs.

Hantaviruses

The hantaviruses are also part of the family *Bunyaviridae,* but comprise a recently recognized genus (Schmaljohn and Dalrymple, 1983). The name of the type species, Hantaan virus, and the genus name, *Hantavirus*, come from the Hantaan River in the demilitarized zone between North and South Korea, where the rodent that yielded the original Hantaan virus isolate was captured in 1976. Until recently, there were three major hantaviruses associated with human disease: Hantaan virus, which is found primarily in Asia and was first isolated from the striped field mouse, *Apodemus agrarius;* Seoul virus, first isolated from Norway rats; and Puumala virus, which was isolated from bank voles and is found mainly in Europe (reviewed in McKee et al., 1991). These hantaviruses cause a disease called hemorrhagic fever with renal syndrome (HFRS) (McKee et al., 1985), and their global impact on health is substantial. In China, well over 100,000 hospitalized HFRS cases occur annually, with a mortality rate of approximately 5%. There is evidence to suggest that the endemic region of Hantaan virus in China is spreading to the south, with increasingly large areas involved (Yu-tu, 1983). Similar, though less severe, forms of HFRS occur in Europe (known locally as nephropathia epidemica), and there is growing evidence of human hantavirus infection in many other parts of the world (LeDuc et al., 1986; Lee, 1993).

Although relatively few data are available, infection of the natural rodent host with any of the hantaviruses appears to pursue the same course: a transient viremia is followed by a brisk neutralizing antibody response that coincides with the termination of viremia; in spite of the presence of circulating neutralizing antibody, there is prolonged and persistent viruria, as well as virus shedding in saliva and feces (Lee et al., 1981). Chronic viremic infection is not believed to occur, and the mechanism of the persistent excretion of virus in urine, feces, and saliva remains ill-defined. Hantaviruses are readily transmitted by the aerosol route (Nuzum et al., 1988), and humans are thought to be infected primarily by aerosol. There are several dramatic examples of persons becoming infected following very brief visits to animal rooms where infected rodents were kept (Tsai, 1987; LeDuc, 1987). Transmission between rodents may occur by aerosol or perhaps more commonly by bite (Childs et al., 1994; Childs et al., 1988; Glass et al., 1988).

Seoul virus was first discovered in Seoul, Korea, when an apartment house resident became ill with a disease similar to classic HFRS (formerly called Korean hemorrhagic fever), which at that time was associated only with Hantaan virus infection. Epidemiologic investigations found no history of travel to known Hantaan virus–endemic areas, but the man had recently been bitten by an urban rat *(Rattus norvegicus),* which he subsequently killed with a broomstick. Rodent collections in the apartment failed to capture any *A. agrarius.* However, Norway rats were common, and when examined serologically, these rats were found to have antibodies that reacted with Hantaan virus (Lee et al., 1982). The hypothesis was then proposed that urban rodents had become infected with Hantaan virus, and that perhaps these rodents had been distributed throughout the world by international shipping. In response to this idea, rodents were captured from several sites, and in virtually every location where rodents were abundant, evidence was also found of hantavirus infection (LeDuc et al., 1984; Tsai et al., 1985; LeDuc et al., 1986). Only after careful laboratory examination was it determined that the viruses isolated from domestic rats were distinct from classic Hantaan virus, and the name Seoul virus was proposed. Subsequent studies have now shown that the ratborne hantaviruses have similar neutralization test reactions, have a genetic similarity of more than 96%, and are highly conserved at the amino acid level (Chu et al., 1993; Arthur et al., 1992; Xiao et al., 1993).

The Norway rat, *R. norvegicus,* is the primary host of Seoul virus. This species originated in Asia and has spread worldwide in relatively recent times. For example, the species probably did not reach Britain until the early 1700s. It was not identified in Montana, United States, until 1923. The wide distribution of these rat viruses, and their similarity, is very strong evidence that they were originally distributed with the rats. It is important that Seoul virus is genetically more closely related to Hantaan virus another virus of murid rodents (Chu et al., 1993) (Table 5, Fig. 1). Thus, phylogenetic relationships of the viruses are congruent to those of their rodent hosts, an important theme in the molecular evolution of hantaviruses and arenaviruses.

In the summer of 1993, a new hantaviral disease—hantavirus pulmonary syndrome (HPS)—appeared dramatically in the southwestern United States (Nichol et al., 1993; Ksiazek et al., 1995; Duchin et al., 1994; Butler and Peters, 1994). This newly recognized infection was caused by a hantavirus carried by the deer mouse, *Peromyscus maniculatus* (Childs et al., 1994) and has now been identified in 21 different states (CDC, 1993a; CDC, 1994a). A febrile prodrome with constitutional symptoms is followed by the abrupt onset of noncardiogenic pulmonary edema and shock, with death ensuing in more than half the identified patients. Serologic evidence demonstrated the hantaviral etiology, reverse transcriptase and polymerase chain reaction assays yielded genetic information that permitted the identification of the agent as a novel hantavirus, and immunohistochemical antigen tracing provided the pathophysiological link that made the implication of a virus from a genus so closely associated with renal disease plausible. Indeed, a few cases of HFRS appear to have more extensive pulmonary involvement early in their course (Giles et al., 1954).

The investigation that led to the elucidation of the disease syndrome and the rapid identification of its causative agent was possible only through coordinated interaction of multiple agencies, the application of modern techniques in molecular biology, and the presence of an experienced infrastructure at CDC (Hughes et al., 1993). This approach illustrates the type of effort that should be mounted against emerging or

Table 10.5. *Some rodent hosts, their viruses, and their taxonomic affinities*

	RODENT	COMMON NAME	VIRUS
Murid	*Rattus norvegicus*	Norway rat	Seoul
	Apodemus agrarius	Striped field mouse	Hantaan
	Mus musculus	House mouse	Lymphocytic choriomeningitis
	Mastomys species	Multimammate mouse	Lassa
Sigmodontine (formerly Cricetine)	*Peromyscus maniculatus*	Deer mouse	Sin Nombre[a]
	Sigmodon hispidus	Cotton rat	Black Creek Canal; Tamiami
	Calomys callosus	"laucha"	Machupo
	Calomys musculinus	"laucha"	Junin
	Sigmodon alstoni	Cotton rat	Guanarito
Microtine or Arvicolid	*Clethrionomys glareolus*	Bank vole	Puumala[a]
	Microtus pennsylvanicus	Meadow vole	Prospect Hill[a]

[a]These viruses are hantaviruses; the remainder are arenaviruses.

introduced hemorrhagic fevers and other microbial threats (CDC, 1994b).

After considerable difficulty, the causative virus, initially called Muerto Canyon virus but now definitively named Sin Nombre virus, was finally isolated in a tractable form in cell culture (Elliot et al., 1994). Preliminary results suggest that this new group of hantaviruses shares the same persistence characteristics as those attributed to other better known

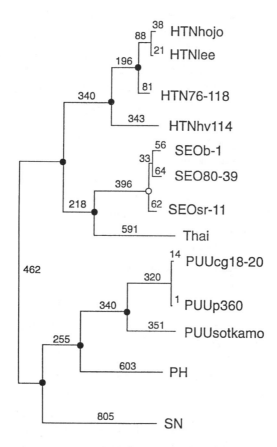

Figure 1 Phylogenetic relationship of Sin Nombre virus relative to previously characterized hantaviruses. Phylogenetic analysis of the complete M segment (3696 bases) aligned hantavirus nucleotide sequences was carried out by the maximum parsimony method using PAUP software. A single most parsimonious tree was obtained. Bootstrap confidence limits in excess of 50% are indicated at appropriate branch points. Limits of 100% are indicated by closed circles and a limit of 50% is indicated by an open circle. Horizontal lengths are proportional to nucleotide step differences (indicated adjacent to line). Vertical distances are for graphic representation only.

members of the genus. The virus appears to persist in chronically infected deer mice, in which it is likely to be shed into the environment by way of infectious urine, feces, and saliva. This assumption is supported by the detection of viral nucleic acid in tissues of virtually all seropositive mice examined. As with other hantaviruses, the true mechanism of spread between rodents and to humans is unproven, but anecdotal observations on individual cases of HPS suggest that transmission to humans is similar to that of other hantaviruses and is most likely via the aerosol route. The virus probably persists in nature within the rodent population, and because of ecological conditions, rodent populations in the southwestern United States were able to reach tenfold or greater their normal densities in the spring and early summer of 1993 (Parmenter et al., 1993), leading to increased exposure of humans to potentially infected deer mice and the subsequent appearance of the outbreak.

As a result of national surveillance for HPS, two additional species of previously unrecognized hantaviruses have recently been identified from human tissues or rodents in the United States (CDC, 1993a; CDC, 1994b). One of these has been isolated from a cotton rat and named Black Creek Canal virus. At present, the global distribution of viruses capable of causing HPS is unknown, although preliminary results suggest that such disease may occur in Brazil and Argentina (Nichol et al., 1994; Parisi et al., 1992). Interestingly, the viruses associated to date with HPS form a genetic group and are more closely related to each other than to the hantaviruses from microtine rodents, such as Prospect Hill or Puumala viruses, or to those from murid rodents, such as Hantaan or Seoul viruses (Table 5, Figure 1) The two established reservoirs of viruses that cause HPS, deer mice and cotton rats, are both sigmodontine (or cricetine) rodents. This observation suggests the testable hypothesis that the sigmodontine-derived viruses are likely to cause HPS rather than HFRS. If so, HPS will be mainly a disease of the Americas because sigmodontines are widely distributed and numerous in North and South America and their closest relatives are mainly represented elsewhere by various species of hamsters.

Arenaviruses

Viruses of the family *Arenaviridae* use different mechanisms of persistence but are maintained in nature virtually exclusively by chronic infections of rodents (Childs and Peters, 1993). Arenaviruses were serologically grouped into those found in the New World and those from the Old World and there is a genetic basis for this grouping, (Clegg, 1993). Human pathogenic arenaviruses from the New World include Junin virus, cause of Argentine hemorrhagic fever; Machupo virus, cause of Bolivian hemorrhagic fever; Guanarito virus, cause of Venezuelan hemorrhagic fever; and Sabia virus, cause of a newly recognized hemorrhagic disease seen only in a fatal case resident near Sao Paulo, Brazil (Coimbra et al., 1994). Subsequent Sabia virus infections have occurred in two laboratory workers in Brazil and the United States, attesting to the aerosol infectivity of arenaviruses (CDC, 1993b). Other arenaviruses have been found in the Americas, but they have not been associated with significant human illness. Interestingly, one of these, Tamiami virus, is also associated with the cotton rat host of Black Creek Canal hantaviruses (Table 5). The only Old World arenavirus causing hemorrhagic fever is Lassa virus from West Africa. Lymphocytic choriomeningitis (LCM) virus is now found virtually worldwide as a consequence of the migrations of its rodent host, the house mouse. LCM virus does not cause hemorrhagic manifestations, but it is responsible for central nervous system syndromes (Peters, 1994) and congenital hydrocephalus (Barton et al., 1993) in humans.

As with hantaviruses, it is of interest to examine the taxonomy of the rodents that are involved in the maintenance of these viruses. All the New World arenaviruses are associated with sigmodontine rodents. Both Lassa and LCM viruses cause chronic infections of murid rodents. In the case of LCM virus, both the rodent *(Mus musculus)* and the virus originated in the Old World, but were introduced into the New World in post-Columbian times. The mouse and its viral parasite are found virtually everywhere investigators have attempted to look in both North and South America, suggesting a very ancient viral accompaniment of *M. musculus* in its travels. There is a strong resemblance to the movements of Seoul virus with *Rattus norvegicus*.

Lassa fever is a major public health problem in West Africa, with many thousands of cases and probably thousands of deaths annually. It is responsible for an important proportion of patients admitted to hospital wards. This virus is maintained by a common African rodent, *Mastomys,* that is well adjusted to living in close association with humans. Rodents of this genus actually represent a species complex; related species are distributed widely over the continent. Some other Old World arenaviruses of unknown public health importance also infect *Mastomys,* but will not be discussed here.

Several factors contribute to the pattern of persistent infection in these animals, which results in the continued maintenance of Lassa virus in endemic foci of Africa. If newborns are infected, they all develop viremia, leading to viruria, and these continue indefinitely (Murphy and Walker, 1978). That is, they become chronically infected, shedding infectious virus into the environment and potentially infecting susceptible humans, for their entire life. Elsewhere in this book the mechanism behind persistent arenavirus infection with LCM virus is discussed by Rafi Ahmed. Animals that are more than two weeks of age when infected, however, show a different response pattern. They all develop viremia, but it is short-lived. They synthesize antibodies and apparently clear the infection. This is exactly the same pattern that is seen with LCM virus and house mice.

While this persistent infection in a proportion of the rodents may maintain the virus for the life of the rodent, it does not resolve the question of long-term, intergenerational maintenance. If newborn infected animals that are persistently viremic are bred, they are normally fertile, and all their offspring will be infected, thus offering a tightly linked, congenital, intergenerational transmission of the virus that ensures persistence in nature. Animals infected later in life have a transient viremia, followed by development of cellular responses that clear the infection. These animals will produce offspring that are born without viral infection but with maternal antibody that protects them from early infection. These newborns will be weaned uninfected; if infected later in life, they will experience an infection that again does not lead to chronicity. Thus, adult infection with these viruses probably leads to a dead end with regard to long term persistence of the infection in nature. While some virus is shed, it probably is insignificant in terms of the overall maintenance of the virus.

Chronic infection with Old World arenaviruses appears to have little or no impact on the rodent host. Available data on infected animals usually show normal growth and fertility. Descriptions of immunopathology related to LCM in mice are largely irrelevant to the natural maintenance because laboratory strains of virus and inbred strains of mice were selected.

Persistence mechanisms among the New World arenaviruses are more complex. Those associated with human disease are very focal in nature, and generally are uniquely associated with a single species of rodent host. The mechanism of regulation of spread of the New World arenaviruses is not known, but it is clear from examination of Junin virus, the cause of Argentine hemorrhagic fever, that this disease is invading new areas each year. It first appeared in the 1950s in a small focus in the Argentine pampas and has subsequently expanded until it is now widely distributed through this rich farming region (Maiztegui and Sabattini, 1977). It is difficult to envision the long-term consequence of this spread: that is, whether it will continue to spread, contract, or disappear. The key to the spread may be related to the mechanism by which these viruses are maintained in the host.

Unlike LCM virus and house mice, persistence of New World arenaviruses, such as Junin and Machupo viruses, is not a tightly linked congenital process. All newborn rodents that are infected become viremic; however, adult infection results in approximately half of the animals becoming viremic, and half clearing their viremia and developing neutralizing antibodies. A major difference between the New World arenaviruses and LCM virus in their respective rodent hosts is that there is strongly reduced reproductive success among inseminated rodents chronically viremic with Junin or Machupo viruses. Thus, the rodents do not contribute to the intergenerational transfer of the virus in nature, although they certainly do contribute to human disease through excretion of virus into the environment. Indeed, field studies suggest a dominant role for horizontal transmission in the spread of virus among rodents and risk to humans in endemic zones (Mills et al., 1994). In the case of Machupo virus infection, those adult female rodents whose original infection was cleared remain fertile, with their offspring protected by maternal antibody. When an uninfected female is mated with an infected male, infected offspring are produced. The female becomes infected at the time of breeding and will produce offspring that are infected. At her next breeding, she will either be chronically viremic, in which case we expect virtually all her embryos to die, or she will have cleared her viremia and will protect her offspring through maternal antibody. Thus, as rodent populations rise there is an increased opportunity for contact and spreading infection, but the infection may also be sterilizing in a proportion of rodents. There has been speculation that this might serve as an oscillating system of natural checks and balances to ensure that both the virus and the rodent hosts persist (Webb et al., 1975).

Crimean Congo hemorrhagic fever and flaviviruses

Both these arthropod-borne viruses grow in cultures of cells from the respective arthropod hosts without causing cytopathic effect and chronically infect their arthropod vector. Crimean Congo hemorrhagic fever is a member of the family *Bunyaviridae*, genus *Nairovirus,* and is transmitted by *Hyalomma* ticks between vertebrate hosts (Peters and LeDuc, 1991; Camicas, et al., 1994). The virus successfully survives in the ticks as they mature through the development of larvae and nymph to adult. There is also transovarial transmission to the next generation of ticks, but the relative efficiency and importance are not known in detail (Gonzalez et al., 1992).

Yellow fever (family *Flaviviridae*) is usually transmitted from vertebrate to vertebrate by chronically infected mosquitoes, but intergenerational transfer is not thought to be quantitatively important. Nevertheless, vertical transmission of yellow fever virus has been shown in the laboratory (Dutary and LeDuc, 1981; Aitken et al., 1979) and suggested from field material (Cornet et al., 1979). With yellow fever and other flaviviruses vertical transmission occurs, not transovarially, but rather at the time of oviposition (Rosen, 1988). Recognition of this mechanism may lead to further understanding of its importance in yellow fever maintenance.

Implications for filoviruses

The search for the natural reservoir of the filoviruses has been vigorous since their initial recognition in 1967, but has not been successful. Comparison to other hemorrhagic fever viruses (Table 4) would suggest that filoviruses may well have a mammalian reservoir in which a chronic infection is established. Filoviruses, like arenaviruses, are relatively insensitive to the antiviral action of interferon and also produce only slight to moderate cytopathic effect in mammalian cell lines. All the other viruses in Table 2 are readily neutralized by convalescent-phase sera *in vitro* with the exception of Lassa virus. Recovery from filovirus infections and Lassa virus infections appears to depend on presumably cellular effector mechanisms other than humoral immunity. In addition, the filoviruses contain a putatively immunosuppressive amino acid motif that may be active in mammalian systems (Volchkov et al., 1992; Peters et al., 1994), and arenaviruses produce immunosuppressive variants after infection (Ahmed, this volume). These comparisons prove nothing, but taken together suggest that examination of mammalian hosts for chronic filovirus infection must be a continuing priority in the search for the elusive natural reservoir of Marburg and Ebola viruses.

Conclusions

The hemorrhagic fever viruses (Table 2) are relatively simple RNA viruses that appear to depend on chronic infection as a link in their natural transmission cycle to assure their persistence in nature (Table 4). In addition, there is often a specific mechanism that leads to intergenerational propagation. In the case of most arenaviruses and RVF virus, this appears to be an important feature of the natural history of the virus. In the case of Crimean-Congo hemorrhagic fever, yellow fever, and some arenaviruses, the link between the two generations is nonconstant and may only serve as a back–up mechanism. No element of vertical transmission has been identified among hantaviruses.

There is generally a non-cytopathic interaction with cells derived from the persistently infected host (Table 3). In the case of arenaviruses, insensitivity to interferon and immunosuppression play a role in chronic viremic infections of their rodent hosts. With hantaviruses, there appears to be a normal systemic immune response, but long-term mucosal virus shedding occurs to assure persistence via infection of native rodents.

Bibliography

Aitken, T. H. G., Tesh, R. B., Beaty, B. J., et al. (1979). Transovarial transmission of yellow fever virus by mosquitos (Aedes aegypti). Am. J. Trop. Med. Hyg. 28:119–121.

Arthur, R. R., Lofts, R. S., Glass, G. E., LeDuc, J. W. and Childs, J. E. (1992). Grouping of hantaviruses by the PCR amplification of S genome segment using consensus primers. Am. J. Trop. Med. Hyg. 47:210–224.

Barton, L. L., Budd, S. C., Morfitt, W. S., Peters, C. J., Ksiazek, T. G., Schindler, R. F., and Yoshino, M. T. (1993). Congenital lymphocytic choriomeningitis virus infection in twins. Pediatr. Infect. Dis. J. 12:942–946.

Battles, J. K. and Dalrymple, J. M. (1988). Genetic variation among geographic isolates of Rift Valley fever virus. Am. J. Trop. Med. Hyg. 39:617–631.

Butler, J. C., and Peters, C. J. (1994). Hantaviruses and hantavirus pulmonary syndrome. Clin. Infect. Dis. 19:387–395.

Camicas, J. L., Cornet, J. D., Gonzalez, J. P., Wilson, M. L., Adam, F., and Zeller, H. G. (1994). Crimean-Congo hemorrhagic fever in Senegal: present status of the knowledge on the ecology of the CCHF virus. Bull. Soc. Pathol. Exot. 87:11–16.

CDC. (1993a). Hantavirus pulmonary syndrome—Virginia, 1993. M.M.W.R. 43:876–877.

CDC. (1994b). Addressing emerging infectious disease threats: a prevention strategy for the United States. Public Health Service, Department of Health and Human Services, Atlanta, Georgia.

CDC. (1994a). Newly identified hantavirus—Florida, 1994. M.M.W.R. 43:99,105.

CDC. (1993b). Arenavirus infection—Connecticut, 1994. M.M.W.R. 43:635.

Childs, J. E., Glass, G. E., Korch, G. W., and LeDuc, J. W. (1988). The ecology and epizootiology of hantaviral infections in small mammal communities of Baltimore: A review and synthesis. Bull. Soc. Vector Ecol. 13:113–122.

Childs, J. E., Ksiazek, T. G., Spiropoulou, C. F., et al., (1994). Serologic and genetic identification of Peromyscus maniculatus as the primary reservoir for a new hantavirus in the southwestern United States. J. Infect. Dis. 169:1271–1280.

Childs, J. C., and Peters, C. J. (1993). Ecology and epidemiology of arenaviruses and their hosts. In: The Arenaviridae. Salvato, M. S. (Editor), Plenum Press, New York, 331–373.

Chu, Y. C., Rossi, C. A., LeDuc, J. W., Lee, H. W., Schmaljohn, C. S., and Dalrymple, J. M. (1993). Serological relationships among viruses in the Hantavirus genus, family Bunyaviridae. Virology 198:196–204.

Clegg, J. C. S., (1993). Molecular phylogeny of the arenaviruses and guide to published sequence data. In: The Arenaviridae. Salvato, M. S. (Editor), Plenum Press, New York, 175–187.

Coimbra, L. T. M., Nassar, E. S., and Burattini, M. N., et al. (1994). New arenavirus isolated in Brazil. *Lancet 343*:391–392.

Cornet, M., Robin, Y., Heme, G., et al. (1979). Une poussee epizootique de fievre jaune selvatique du Senegal oriental: isolement du virus de lots de moustiques adultes et femelles. *Med. Malad. Infect. 9*:63–66

Davies, F. G., Linthicum, K. J., and James, A. D. (1985). Rainfall and epizootic Rift Valley fever. *Bull. W.H.O. 63*:941–943.

Duchin, J. S., Koster, F., Peters, C. J., et al. (1994). Hantavirus pulmonary syndrome: a clinical description of 17 patients with a newly recognized disease. *N. Engl. J. Med. 330*:949–955.

Dutary, B. E., and LeDuc, J. W. (1981). Transovarial transmission of yellow fever virus by a sylvatic vector, *Haemogogus equinus. Trans. R. Soc. Trop. Med. Hyg. 75*:128.

Elliot, L. H., Ksiazek, T. G., Rollin, P. E., et al. (1994). Isolation of the causative agent of hantavirus pulmonary syndrome. *Am. J. Trop. Med. Hyg. 51*:102–105.

Faran, M. E., Romoser, W. S., Routier, R. G., and Bailey, C. L. (1986). Use of the avidin–biotin–peroxidase complex immunocytochemical procedure for detection of Rift Valley fever virus in paraffin sections of mosquitoes. *Am. J. Trop. Med. Hyg. 35*:1061–1067.

Faran, M. E., Romoser, W. S., Routier, R. G., and Bailey, C. L. (1988). The distribution of Rift Valley fever virus in the mosquito *Culex pipiens* as revealed by viral titration of dissected organs and tissues. *Am. J. Trop. Med. Hyg. 39*:206–213.

Giles, R. B., Sheedy, J. A., Ekman, C. N., et al. (1954). The sequelae of epidemic hemorrhagic fever with a note on causes of death. *Am. J. Med. 16*:629–638.

Glass, G. E., Childs, J. E., Korch, G. W., and LeDuc, J. W. (1988). Association of intraspecific wounding with hantaviral infection in wild rats *(Rattus norvegicus). Epidemiol. Infect. Dis. 101*:459–472.

Gonzales, J. P., Camicas, J. L., Cornet, J. P., Faye, O., and Wilson, M. L. (1992). Sexual and transovarian transmission of Crimean-Congo haemorrhagic fever virus in *Hyalomma truncatum* ticks. *Res. Virol. 143*:23–28.

Hughes, J. M., Peters, C. J., Cohen, M. L., and Mahy, B. W. J. (1993). Hantavirus pulmonary syndrome: An emerging infectious disease. *Science 262*:850–851.

Ksiazek, T. G., Peters, C. J., Rollin, P. E., et al. (1995). Identification of a new North American hantavirus that causes acute pulmonary insufficiency. *Am. J. Trop. Med. 52*:117–123.

LeDuc, J. W. (1979). The ecology of California group viruses. *J. Med. Entomol. 16*:1–17.

LeDuc, J. W. (1987). Epidemiology of Hantaan and related viruses. *Lab. Anim. Sci. 37*:413–418.

LeDuc, J. W., Smith, G. A., Childs, J. E., et al. (1986). Global survey of antibody to Hantaan related viruses among peridomestic rodents. *Bull. W.H.O. 64*:139–144.

LeDuc, J. W., Smith, G. A., and Johnson, K. M. (1984). Hantaan-like viruses from domestic rats captured in the United States. *Am. J. Trop. Med. Hyg. 33*:992–998.

Lee, H. W. (1993). *Global distribution of hemorrhagic fever with renal syndrome and hantaviruses*. In: Concepts in virology. Mahy, B. W. J. and Lvov, D. I. (Editors). Harwood Academic Press, Chur, Switzerland, 299–307.

Lee, H. W., Baek, L. J. and Johnson, K. M. (1982). Isolation of Hantaan virus, the etiologic agent of Korean hemorrhagic fever, from wild urban rats. *J. Infect. Dis.* *146*:638–644.

Lee, H. W., Lee, P. W., Baek, L. J., Song, C. K., and Seong, I. W. (1981). Intraspecific transmission of Hantaan virus, etiologic agent of Korean hemorrhagic fever, in the rodent *Apodemus agrarius*. *Am. J. Trop. Med. Hyg. 30*:1106–1112.

Linthicum, K. J., Bailey, C. L., Tucker, C. J., et al. (1991). Towards real-time prediction of Rift Valley fever epidemics in Africa. *J. Prevent. Vet. Med. 11*:325–334.

Linthicum, K. J., Davies, F. G., Kairo, A., and Bailey, C. L. (1985). Rift Valley fever virus (Family *Bunyaviridae*, genus *Phlebovirus*). Isolations from Diptera collected during an interepizootic period in Kenya. *J. Hyg. 95*:197–209.

Logan, T. M., Linthicum, K. J., Wagateh, J. N., Thande, P. C., Kamau, C. W., and Roberts, C. R. (1990). Pretreatment of floodwater *Aedes* habitats (dambos) in Kenya with a sustained-release formulation of methoprene. *J. Am. Mosq. Control Assoc.* *6*:736–738.

Maiztegui, J. I., and Sabattini, M. S. (1977). Extension progresiva del area endemica de fiebre hemorrhagica Argentina. *Medicine (Buenos Aires) 37*:162–166.

McKee, K. T., Jr., LeDuc, J. W., and Peters, C. J. (1991). *Hantaviruses*. In: The textbook of human virology, 2nd Ed. Belshe, R. B. (Editor), 615–632.

McKee, K. T., MacDonald, C., LeDuc, J. W. and Peters, C. J. (1985). Hemorrhagic fever with renal syndrome. *Mil. Med. 150*:640–647.

Mills, J. N., Ellis, B. A., Childs, J. E., et al. (1994). Prevalence of infection with Junin virus in rodent populations in the epidemic area of Argentine hemorrhagic fever. *Am. J. Trop. Med. Hyg. 51*:554–562.

Murphy, F. A., and Walker, D. H. (1978). *Arenaviruses: Persistent infection and viral survival in reservoir hosts*. In: Virus and environment. Kurstak, E. and Maramorosch, K. (Editors), Academic Press, New York, 155–180.

Nichol, S. T., Morzunov, S., Chizhikov, V., et al. (1994). Abstract: Of mice and men: hantavirus genetics and pulmonary syndrome. *Ninth International Conference on Negative Strand Viruses*, October 2–7, 1994.

Nichol, S. T., Spiropoulou, C. F., Morzunov, S. et al. (1993). Genetic identification of a hantavirus associated with an outbreak of acute respiratory illness. *Science* *262*:914–917.

Nuzum, E. O., Rossi, C. A., Stephenson, E. H. and LeDuc, J. W. (1988). Aerosol transmission of Hantaan and related viruses to laboratory rats. *Am. J. Trop. Med. Hyg.* *38*:636–640.

Parisi, M. N., Tiano, E., Enria, D., Sabattini, M., and Maiztegui, J. I. (1992). Actividad de un hantavirus en pacientes de la zona endemica de Fiebre Hemorragica Argentina (FHA). *Fourteenth Annual Reunion of the Argentine Society of Virology*, Buenos Aires, 10–11 December 1992.

Parmenter, R. R., Brunt, J. W., Moore, D. I., and Ernest, S. (1993). *The hantavirus epidemic in the Southwest: rodent population dynamics and the implications for transmission of hantavirus-associated adult respiratory distress syndrome (HARDS) in the Four Corners region.* Albuquerque (NM): University of New Mexico, Department of Biology; July. Sevilleta LTER Publication No. 41.

Peters, C. J. (1994). *Arenavirus infections.* In: Handbook of neurovirology. McKendall, R. R. and Stroop, W. G., (Editors), Marcell Dekker, New York, 621–637.

Peters, C. J. (1996). *Hemorrhagic fevers.* In: Nathanson, N. (Editor) Viral pathogenesis. Raven Press, New York, in press.

Peters, C. J. and Anderson, G. W. (1981). Pathogenesis of Rift Valley fever. In: Goldblum, N., Swartz, T. A., and Klingberg, M. A. (Editors) Contributions to epidemiology and statistics, vol. 3. S. Karger, Basel, 21–41.

Peters, C. J., and LeDuc, J. W. (1991). *Bunyaviridae*: Bunyaviruses, Phleboviruses, and related viruses. In: The textbook of human virology. Belshe, R. B. (Editor), 2nd Edition, 571–614.

Peters, C. J., and Linthicum, K. J. (1994). *Rift Valley fever.* In: Handbook series of zoonoses section B: viral zoonoses,. Beran, G. W. (Editor), CRC Press, Boca Raton, Florida, pp. 125–138.

Peters, C. J., Sanchez, A., Feldman, H., Rollin, P. E., Nichol, S., and Ksiazek, T. G. (1994). Filoviruses as emerging pathogens. *Semin. Virol. 5*:147–154.

Rosen, L. (1988). Further observations on the mechanism of vertical transmission of flaviviruses by *Aedes* mosquitoes. *Am. J. Trop. Med. Hyg. 39*:123–126.

Schmaljohn, C. S., and Dalrymple, J. M. (1983). Analysis of Hantaan virus RNA: evidence for a new genus of *Bunyaviridae*. *Virology 131*:482–491.

Swanepoel, R. (1981). Observations on Rift Valley fever in Zimbabwe. *Contr. Epidem. Biostatist. 3*:83–91.

Tsai, T. F. (1987). Hemorrhagic fever with renal syndrome: Mode of transmission to humans. *Lab. Anim. Sci. 37*:428–430.

Tsai, T. F., Bauer, T. F., and Sasso, D. R. (1985). Serological and virological evidence of a Hantaan virus-related enzootic in the United States. *J. Infect. Dis. 152*:126–136.

Turell, M. J., and Bailey, C. L. (1987). Transmission studies in mosquitoes (Diptera: Culicidae) with disseminated Rift Valley fever virus infections. *J. Med. Entomol. 24*:11–18.

Volchkov, V. E., Blinov, V. M., and Netesov, S. V. (1992). The envelope glycoprotein of Ebola virus contains an immunosuppressive-like domain similar to oncogenic retroviruses. *FEBS Lett. 305*:181–184.

Webb, P. A., Justines, G., and Johnson, K. M. (1975). Infection of wild and laboratory animals with Machupo and Latino viruses. *Bull. W.H.O. 52*:493–500.

Xiao, S.-Y., LeDuc, J. W., Chu, Y. K., and Schmaljohn, C. S. (1993). Phylogenetic analyses of virus isolates in the genus *Hantavirus*, family *Bunyaviridae*. *Virology 198*:205–217.

Yu-tu, J. (1983). A preliminary report on hemorrhagic fever with renal syndrome in China. *Chin. Med. J. 96*:265–268.

11

Anti-viral CD8+ cytotoxic T cell memory

Lisa L. Lau and Rafi Ahmed*
Department of Microbiology and Immunology
UCLA School of Medicine
Los Angeles, CA 90024, USA

Introduction

The enhanced response of the immune system upon second exposure to an antigen is a central concept of immunology and the basis of vaccination against infectious diseases. Protective anti-viral immunity, often lasting several decades, occurs in many natural infections, and many of the currently used live vaccines confer long-term immunity. Less clear is how immunological memory is generated and then maintained after a viral infection is controlled. While there is a fair amount in the literature about antibody responses following these natural infections and vaccinations, much less is known about cytotoxic T lymphocyte (CTL) activation and memory (Mackay, 1992; Ahmed, 1992; Beverley, 1990; Cerottini et al., 1989; Celada, 1971). Acute infection of adult mice with lymphocytic choriomeningitis virus (LCMV) provides a useful experimental system to study these aspects of CTL differentiation. In this model, viral clearance occurs within two to four weeks after infection and is mediated in large part by a potent primary CTL response. Thereafter, the mice are protected for their lifespan against reinfection with the original infecting strain and more virulent strains of the virus (Ahmed, 1984). This protection is me-

---

*Now at Department of Microbiology, Emory University, Atlanta, GA 30322, USA

diated by memory CTL (Jamieson and Ahmed, 1989). Using the LCMV model, we have been able to compare effector and memory CTL and naive, unprimed cells, both quantitatively and phenotypically. We have also addressed questions regarding the requirements for long-term maintenance of CTL memory. In particular, we have examined the dependence of CTL memory on persistent antigenic stimulation. For B cells, a widely held view is that the original antigen, trapped in immune complexes on follicular dendritic cells, provides continuous stimulation of specific memory cells (Tew et al., 1980; Klaus et al., 1980). We asked whether the same is true for memory CTL. Using adoptive transfer into uninfected recipients, we assessed the *in vivo* survival of memory CD8+ CTL in a specific antigen-free environment. Adoptively transferred anti-viral CTL were found to persist indefinitely in the absence of priming antigen and to confer protection against virus challenge (Lau et al., 1994). The results reviewed in this chapter provide evidence for the existence of memory CTL that are not dependent on specific antigen for their survival, thus invoking different mechanisms of maintaining memory within the immune system.

Results And Discussion

Direct ex vivo *measurement of the primary CTL response in an acute LCMV infection*

Virus-specific CTL activity in the spleen can be detected in ^{51}Cr release assays (Fig. 1A) by day 5 after intraperitoneal (i.p.) or intravenous (i.v.) infection of adult mice with the Armstrong strain of LCMV. Before this timepoint, target cell lysis is non-specific and mediated by natural killer cells. The primary CTL response is rapid and peaks at day 8 post-infection. Its effect is easily discerned because levels of infectious virus in the spleen drop more than 4 logs between day 3 and day 8 after infection (Fig. 1B). In addition, the potent primary CTL response in the spleen prevents widespread viral dissemination to other tissues. By day 15, viral titers in the spleen and serum are below detection in standard plaque assays. In parallel with the elimination of infection, spleen CTL activity, measured in direct *ex vivo* assays, declines to baseline levels by day 20 to 30.

In contrast, anti-LCMV antibody levels measured in the serum are first detectable at around day 5 and remain high for the lifespan of the immunized animal. Because the effector phase of the CTL response to an acute LCMV infection is short-lived, and similar transient responses have been observed in other acute viral infections, it has been suggested that CTL memory does not exist (Zinkernagel, 1990). However, while the direct ^{51}Cr release assay measures lytic activity in a bulk population of cells, it does not indicate the actual number of CTL present among those cells. In fact, primed, memory CTL can be distinguished from naive CD8+ T lymphocytes by their frequency in virus-immune mice. Limiting dilution analysis of LCMV-specific CTL precursors (CTLp) shows that memory CTL are long-lived and differ quantitatively from naive T cells.

Quantitation of LCMV-specific CTL precursors following immunization

At various timepoints after a primary infection of adult H-2^b mice, the frequency of LCMV-specific CTLp was determined by limiting dilution analysis (Fig. 1C). It is important to note that naive lymphocytes could not be primed against LCMV *in vitro* even at high cell concentrations. Between day 0 and day 2 after immunization, the frequency of virus-specific CTL in the spleen is less than 1 in 10^5. In absolute numbers, spleens of uninfected through day 2-infected mice contain less than 10^3 LCMV-specific CTLp. By day 3, however, the frequency rises to 1 in 12,000 spleen cells, equal to about 10^4 specific CTLp. There is massive, exponential expansion of CTL from day 3 to day 8, which corresponds to the striking increase in direct *ex vivo* lytic activity during these timepoints. At day 5, approximately 1 in 380 spleen cells, or about 3.5×10^5 specific CTLp are present. At the peak of the CTL response, the frequency is about 1 in 100, which is about 3×10^6 specific CTLp in absolute numbers. Thus, within 8 days after infection, the number of CTLp specific for LCMV increases about 1000-fold. In Balb/c (H-2^d) mice, the CTL response kinetics are very similar, although the expansion of virus-specific CTLp between day 0 and day 8 is approximately five-fold less. In the blood, the CTLp frequency curve is almost identical to that of the spleen, but with fewer cells in the circulation.

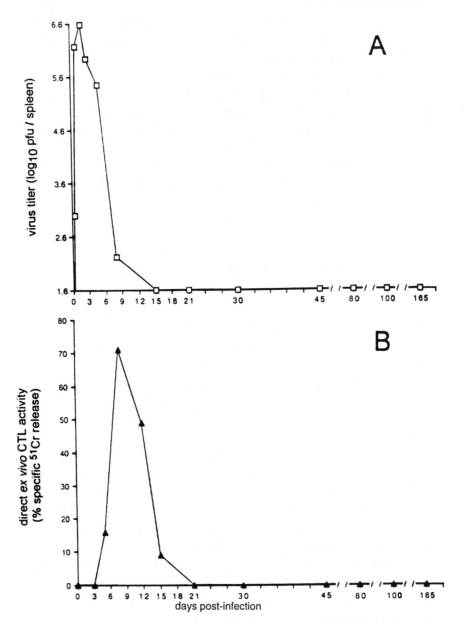

Figure 1 Long-term CTL memory persists following acute LCMV infection.

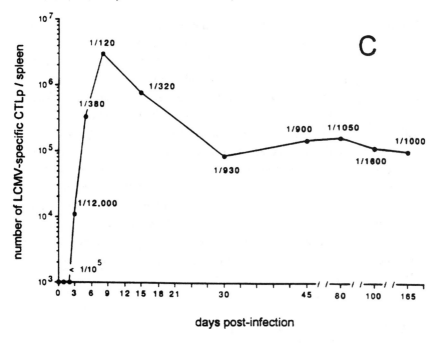

Figure 1 Continued

An interesting event occurs between day 8 and day 30 of the primary CTL response. The majority of CTL, 95 to 98% of the virus-specific effectors measurable at day 8, will die by apoptosis. It is not entirely clear what induces the cells to die rather than to continue proliferating. Certainly, by day 15, the infection has been controlled and there is no longer abundant antigen presentation to stimulate the dramatic expansion seen early in the CTL response. The decline in CTLp frequency and absolute number mirrors the drop in lytic activity observed in the ^{51}Cr release assay after day 8. However, instead of dropping to baseline levels (less than 1 in 10^5 spleen cells), the frequency of LCMV-specific CTLp stabilizes at about 1 in 1000 in the spleen at day 30 and beyond. In absolute numbers, LCMV-immune mice maintain a stable pool of about 10^5 virus-specific spleen CTLp, which is at least 100-fold higher than in naive mice (Sprent, 1993). Thus, if we look at the CTL response quantitatively dur-

ing the early phase of infection, and then following resolution of infection, we notice that it falls into three phases. There is an initial phase of
expansion, in which there is exponential expansion of the CTL. This is
followed by a phase of death, during which the majority of CTL induced
following primary infection are destined to die. Only about 2 to 5% of
this fraction will survive, and these remain for the lifespan of the animal.
This final phase is one of stability, or memory. One consequence of the
primary viral infection, therefore, is a net increase in the CTL precursor
frequency. However, changes in the surface expression of several adhesion molecules (Bradley et al., 1993; Springer, 1990; Tabi et al., 1988)
indicates that memory CTL also differ qualitatively from naive CD8$^+$ T
lymphocytes. We have focused on the CD44 molecule, which is expressed at low levels on unprimed cells, and at high levels on activated
and memory cells (Stout and Suttles, 1992; MacDonald et al., 1990;
Haynes et al., 1989, Budd et al., 1987).

Polyclonal activation of CD8$^+$ T cells during an acute primary CTL infection

Spleen cells from adult mice were stained by immunofluorescence before
and at various timepoints after acute infection with the Armstrong strain
of LCMV. The cells were stained for either the CD8 or CD4 T cell markers and for CD44. CD44 is also known as Pgp-1 and as Hermes antigen. It
is the receptor for hyaluronate, a component of the extracellular matrix
(Culty et al., 1990; Miyake et al., 1990), and it is believed to be involved
in the adhesion and migration of activated and memory lymphocytes
(Mackay, 1992; Yednock and Rosen, 1989). In unimmunized mice, about
15% of cells in the spleen are CD8$^+$. Within this T cell subset, there are
roughly equal numbers of CD44^{hi} and CD44^{lo} cells. Between day 0 and
day 3 after infection with Armstrong LCMV there is no detectable change
in CD44 expression or in the number of CD8$^+$ T cells in the spleen. However, expansion of the CD8$^+$ subset and doubling of the CD44^{hi} fraction
are noticeable around day 5. At the peak of the CTL response, about 40%
of cells in the spleen are CD8$^+$, and nearly all of these are activated
(CD44^{hi}). What is interesting is that the majority of the CD8$^+$ T cells are
nonspecifically activated. Only about 2 to 5% of these cells are virus-spe-

cific, which means there is fairly extensive polyclonal activation within the CD8$^+$ subset following infection. This is not unique to LCMV. We have observed similar polyclonal activation of CD8$^+$ T cells after infection of mice with vaccinia virus and vesicular stomatitis virus, and using H-2^b or H-2^d mice.

This polyclonal activation is transient and limited to the acute phase of infection. At day 30 and day 90, the CD8$^+$ profile in the spleen is virtually indistinguishable from that of normal, unimmunized mice, although there are slightly more CD8$^+$, CD44^{hi} cells at these timepoints. Thus, the majority of these activated cells, not restricted to virus-specific CTL, die between day 8 and day 30. Based on histology and electron microscopy, the cells appear to die as a result of programmed cell death, or apoptosis. If one looks at spleen sections between day 8 and day 30 it is quite easy to find, within the follicle of the spleen, cells with typical membrane blebs and apoptotic nuclei. This event may be an important and biologically sensible means of maintaining homeostasis in the CD8$^+$ compartment. One would not want an unchecked ten-fold expansion of CD8$^+$ T cells every time one got a viral infection. So there are physiological mechanisms by which most of these cells are eliminated following resolution of an infection.

It is important to point out, however, that while the spleen CD8$^+$ profile from LCMV-immune mice may resemble that of naive, unimmunized mice, the number and frequency of virus-specific CTLp in the former is about 100 times higher than in the latter. We wanted to know whether these cells were CD44^{hi} or CD44^{lo}. Spleen cells from an animal about 90 days post-infection were FACS-sorted into CD44^{hi} (top 30% fluorescent) and CD44^{lo} (bottom 30% fluorescent) fractions. Each fraction contained equal numbers of CD8$^+$ T cells—32% in the CD44^{hi} subset and 26% in the CD44^{lo} subset. LCMV-specific CTLp in each fraction were then quantitated by limiting dilution analysis. The frequency of CD44^{hi}, virus-specific CTLp was 1 in 90 (1.4×10^5 specific CTLp), but the frequency of CD44^{lo}, virus-specific CTLp was 1 in 1.2×10^4 (1.1×10^3 specific CTLp). Thus, nearly all of the long-lived memory CTL segregated with the CD8$^+$, CD44^{hi} phenotype. Memory CTL, therefore, differ quantitatively and qualitatively (phenotypically) from naive cells, and both of these sustained changes contribute to the enhanced secondary immune response.

However, a key, unresolved question is how the properties of long-term memory T cells are maintained. There are two opposing hypotheses regarding this issue. One idea is that long-term T cell immunity is due to long-lived memory cells that can persist in the absence of specific antigen. In this case, the capacity for long-lived T cell survival can be attributed to cells which are distinct from naive cells, and distinct maybe even from primary effector cells. What this suggests is that memory cells are really a separate population of T cells. The second hypothesis is that long-term memory is due to the persistence of the original priming antigen (Zinkernagel, 1993; Gray and Matzinger, 1992; Oehen et al, 1992; Gray and Skarvall, 1988; Feldbush, 1973) in specialized reservoirs, for instance, trapped in immune complexes on follicular epithelial dendritic cells (Klaus et al., 1980; Tew et al., 1980). This persistent antigen would provide continuous, low-level stimulation of primed cells. The issue of antigen persistence is important to resolve, because it is critical in determining how we conceptualize immunological memory and T cell differentiation. Based on our findings, we believe that immune memory, at least for CTL, can be attributed to a distinct group of long-lived cells that do not depend on the continuous presence of the original priming antigen for survival. The studies undertaken to address this topic are described in the next section.

Cytotoxic T cell memory does not require persistent antigenic stimulation

The approach we have used to address whether CTL memory is dependent on persistent antigen has been to adoptively transfer FACS-sorted $CD8^+$ T cells from LCMV-immune mice into naive, uninfected mice, and to assess recovery of donor CTL at various timepoints after transfer. In order to distinguish donor cells from host cells, we used $H\text{-}2^b$ mice congenic at the Thy-1 locus. The donor mice were Thy-1.1^+ (B6.PL-Thy1^a) and the recipient mice were Thy-1.2^+ (C57BL/6). Typically, spleen cells were prepared from LCMV-immune mice 3 months after infection, and $CD8^+$ T cells were isolated by FACS. We were able to obtain a highly purified (>99% pure) population of CD8$^+$ T cells by this method. Cell sorting enabled us to exclude the possibility of antigen-carryover by specialized acessor cells during adoptive transfer. It should be noted as well that the Armstrong strain of LCMV used to immunize the mice does not infect CD8$^+$ T cells. Prior to adoptive transfer, the sorted CD8$^+$ T cells were tested by a number of very sensitive assays for the presence of infectious virus, viral antigen, or viral genetic material. All of these tests were negative. In addition, infectivity tests in which mice were injected with sorted CD8$^+$ cells that had been disrupted by sonication or anti-CD8/C' treatment were also negative. This control rules out the possibility that contaminating virus in the donor CD8$^+$ T cells was being kept in check by active anti-viral CTL. In LCMV, there are three CTL epitopes which are H-2^b-restricted (Whitton et al., 1988). We have carried out PCR to identify these epitopes in the sorted CD8$^+$ T cells from LCMV-immune mice. This analysis did not detect any viral nucleic acid. By quantitative PCR, the sorted CD8$^+$ cells have been found to contain less than one genome equivalent of LCMV per 10^5 cells (data not shown).

2×10^6 FACS-purified CD8$^+$ T cells (Thy-1.1$^+$) from LCMV-immune mice were adoptively transferred into naive, specific antigen-free recipient mice (Thy-1.2$^+$). The precursor frequency of virus-specific CTL in the donor cells was determined by limiting dilution analysis to be about 1 in 100. That meant we had transferred approximately 2×10^4 LCMV-specific CTLp. Following adoptive transfer, the recipient mice were tested routinely for seroconversion. PCR was also performed on spleens from the recipient mice. These tests remained negative at all post-transfer timepoints tested. In addition, the donor CD8$^+$ T cells were unable to stimulate LCMV-specific CTL clones *in vitro* or to prime host T cells *in vivo*. We also checked for a "latent" or low-level infection after adoptive transfer by immunosuppressing the recipient mice. Two adoptive transfer recipients were irradiated (650 rad) about 1 year after receiving 1×10^6 CD8$^+$ T cells from LCMV-immune mice. Prior to irradiation, there was no evidence of infectious virus in the serum, and the mice had not seroconverted. Two weeks after irradiation, the mice were sacrificed, and their tissues (serum, spleen, liver, lung, kidney, and brain) were titrated in plaque assays for the emergence of infectious virus. No infectious virus was detected.

We then asked whether we could recover the donor CTL after parking them in an environment free of any detectable viral material. At regular intervals up to 1 year post-transfer, the recipient mice were sacrificed and their spleen cells were tested for virus-specific CTL in limiting dilution assays (Fig. 2). Initially, about 2×10^4 cells were transferred, and between $5\text{--}10 \times 10^3$ LCMV-specific CTLp were recovered in the spleen up to 12 months post-transfer. Virus-specific CTLp could also be identified in the blood and lymph nodes of the recipient mice, in lower numbers but at similar frequencies. This result demonstrated that memory CTL are not a static population within the spleen, but are continuously circulating, thus fulfilling their role in immune surveillance.

In order to extend our analysis of the survival of memory CTL in the absence of specific antigen, we transferred cells from a group of adoptive recipient mice (18 months post-transfer) into a second batch of uninfected C57BL/6 mice. Each of the 2nd transfer recipients received 2×10^5 Thy-1.1^+ CD8$^+$ cells. LCMV-specific CTLp were quantitated in the input cells at the time of transfer, and in the spleen, lymph nodes, and blood of recipient mice 8 months after the 2nd transfer (the 26-month timepoint). Again, virus-specific CTLp were recovered with little drop in number, and they were found in the circulation as well as in the spleen and lymph nodes.

Memory CTL maintained in the absence of specific antigen retain the CD44^{hi} phenotype

One of the features of long-lived memory CTL in the originally infected mice was their retention of the CD44^{hi} phenotype. We asked whether the CD44^{hi} phenotype was also maintained in the absence of viral antigen. Five months post-transfer, spleen cells from the recipient mice were sorted by FACS into CD44^{hi} (top 30% fluorescent) and CD44^{lo} (bottom 30% fluorescent) fractions. The frequency of LCMV-specific CTLp in each fraction was determined by limiting dilution analysis. All the CTL activity again segregated with the CD44^{hi} subset (Fig. 3). The frequency of donor, LCMV-specific CTLp in this fraction was 1 in 235. The CD44^{lo} fraction, in contrast, had less than 1 in 3×10^3 LCMV-specific CTLp.

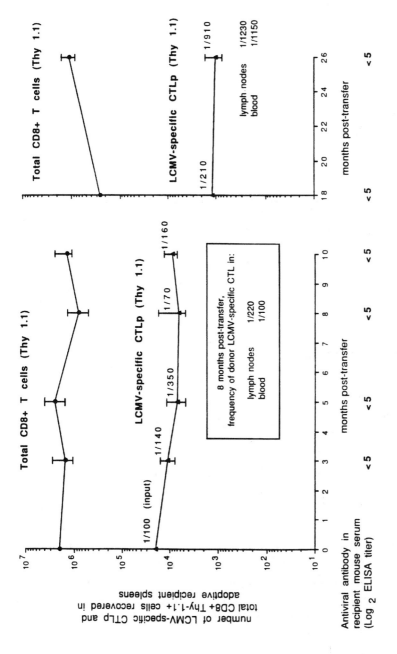

Figure 2 CTL memory persists in the absence of antigen. Quantitation of virus-specific CTLp and total donor CD8⁺ T cells following transfer into uninfected mice.

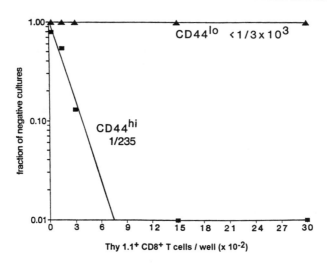

Figure 3 Donor memory CTL parked in uninfected mice retain the CD44hi phenotype.

Memory CTL maintained in the absence of priming antigen are able to protect against reinfection

Thus far, our results provide strong evidence that long-term CTL memory does not wane in the absence of specific antigen. A definitive *in vivo* readout of memory, however, is the ability to protect against reinfection. Therefore, at different times post-transfer, we challenged the adoptive recipients with clone 13, a virulent strain of LCMV (Matloubian et al., 1993; Matloubian et al., 1990; Ahmed et al., 1984). Clone 13 causes a persistent infection in naive adult mice, but is rapidly cleared by immune mice. We reasoned that only the donor memory CTL would be able to control a clone 13 infection, and this would be a good test of their duration in the absence of specific antigen. Three groups of mice which had received sorted CD8+ T cells from LCMV-immune mice were examined. In one group, the donor and recipient mice (H-2b) were congenic at the Thy-1 locus (Thy-1.1 → Thy-1.2). In the second group, both the donor and host mice (H-2b) were completely syngeneic (Thy-1.1 → Thy-1.1). In the third group, we transferred CD8+ T cells from LCMV-immune

Group	Serum virus titers[f] log10pfu / ml (± S.D.)
Thy 1.1 —> Thy 1.2[a]	< 1.7
Thy 1.1 —> Thy 1.1[b]	< 1.7
Thy 1.2[c]	5.16 ± 0.16
Balb/c —> SCID[d]	< 1.7
SCID[e]	5.60 ± 0.23

[a] Uninfected Thy 1.2 mice received 1-2 x 10⁶ CD8+ T cells from LCMV-immune Thy 1.1 mice between 3 and 26 months before Clone 13 challenge.

[b] Uninfected Thy 1.1 mice received 1-2 x 10⁶ CD8+ T cells from syngeneic LCMV-immune Thy 1.1 mice 100 days prior to Clone 13 challenge.

[c] Control, uninfected Thy 1.2 mice.

[d] Uninfected SCID mice received 1-2 x 10⁶ CD8+ T cells from LCMV-immune Balb/c mice 9 months before Clone 13 challenge.

[e] Control, uninfected SCID mice.

[f] Virus titers were measured in plaque assays (Ahmed et al., 1984) 7 days after virus-challenge.

Figure 4 Memory CTL parked in uninfected mice are able to protect against challenge with a virulent strain of LCMV (Clone 13) that causes persistent infection in naive adult mice.

Balb/c (H-2^d) mice into uninfected SCID recipients. Mice from each group of adoptive transfer recipients were challenged with clone 13 and, at various timepoints after infection, we measured viral titers in their sera by plaque assays (Fig. 4). All of these mice, including several challenged 2 years post-transfer, were able to control the clone 13 infection. In contrast, normal H-2^b and H-2^d mice infected with clone 13 were unable to clear the infection, and they became chronically infected with the virus.

Despite the convincing results from these protection experiments, we needed to show that the donor memory CTL were indeed responsible for controlling the clone 13 infection in the adoptive transfer recipients. In this study, we used two C57BL/6 (Thy-1.2) mice which had received 1×10^6 FACS-sorted CD8$^+$ T cells (containing 1×10^4 virus-specific CTLp) from congenic, LCMV-immune B6.PL-Thy-1^a (Thy-1.1) mice. Fifteen months post-transfer, the recipient mice were challenged with clone 13. As controls, normal adult C57BL/6 mice were infected with the same dose of clone 13. Seven days later, virus levels in the spleen and serum were determined by plaque assay, and we measured spleen CTL activity in a ^{51}Cr release assay. In order to distinguish donor and host CTL, we typed the response using allele-specific antibodies to Thy-1 plus C' (Table 1). Normal mice infected with clone 13 were unable to mount a significant CTL response, and the virus replicated to high titers in their spleens and sera. However, both of the adoptive transfer recipients gener-ated a strong CTL response to the clone 13 challenge, which was me-diated entirely by the donor Thy-1.1 cells. Anti-Thy-1.1 antibody/C' completely abrogated the CTL response, while anti-Thy-1.2/C'-treatment had no effect. In addition, viral titers in these mice were below detection in their spleens and sera.

We further characterized the cells responding to viral challenge by double-staining spleen cells from the clone 13-infected transfer recipients with FITC-anti-Thy-1.1 and PE-anti-CD8. The FACS profiles from one of the virus-challenged transfer recipients is shown (Fig. 5). In unchal-lenged transfer recipients, the donor subset comprised about 1 to 2% of total spleen cells (data not shown). However, 7 days after the clone 13 challenge, the donor cells in this recipient had expanded to 17% of total cells in the spleen. The host CD8$^+$ fraction remained unchanged in abso-lute numbers. The two subsets of CD8$^+$ T cells also differed in forward and side scatter, which are cell size and granularity parameters. The host CD8$^+$ cells consisted of a homogeneous population of smaller lympho-cytes (low forward and side scatter). However, the donor CD8$^+$ fraction contained both small and large cells. While no DNA cell-cycle analysis was done on these cells, the data strongly suggest that the large, granular cells are activated lymphoblasts or clusters of CD8$^+$ cells. The selective activation of the donor CD8$^+$ subset makes two important points. First, it shows the dominance of the memory CTL response to viral challenge. Se-

Table 1   *Memory CTL parked in uninfected mice respond to challenge with a virulent strain of LCMV (Clone 13) that causes a persistent infection in naive adult mice*

| Treatment | % Specific ^{51}CR releasee on MC57 (H-2^b) targets | | | | | Virus titer PFU/ml or organ | |
| | LCMV-Infected | | | Uninfected | | | |
	50:1	16.7:1	5.5:1	50:1	16.7:1	Serum	Spleen
Thy 1.1 CD8 → Thy 1.2^a							
recipient 1							
0/C'	47	24	9	1	0	<50	<50
anti-Thy 1.1/C'	3	1	1	2	1		
anti-Thy 1.2/C'	44	18	8	1	0		
recipient 2							
0'C'	63	38	18	1	0	<50	<50
anti-Thy 1.1/C'	2	3	1	1	0		
anti-Thy 1.2/C'	60	37	14	2	0		
Normal Thy 1.2^b							
mouse 1 0/C'	4	3	3	2	0	3.5×10^5	6.5×10^6
mouse 2 0/C'	7	2	0	0	0	8.5×10^4	2.3×10^6

^{a} 1×10^6 FACS-sorted CD8$^+$ T cells (containing 1×10^4 LCMV-specific CTLp) from LCMV-immune Thy 1.1 mice were adoptively transferred into normal Thy 1.2 recipient mice (650 rad). 465 days post-transfer, the recipient mice were challenged with 10^6 pfu Clone 13 LCMV. CTL responses in the spleen and viral titers in the spleen and serum were tested 7 days later.
^{b} Normal Thy 1.2 mice were infected with 10^{6}pfu Clone 13 LCMV at the same time the transfer recipients were challenged. Spleen CTL responses and viral titers in the spleen and serum were checked after 7 days.

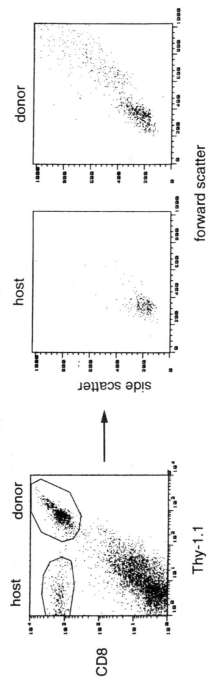

Figure 5 Proliferation of parked memory CTL after re-exposure to virus. Phenotypic analysis and cell size analysis by FACS.

cond, it provides further evidence that host CTL were not primed by the LCMV-immune donor cells.

Conclusion

The major finding of our studies on cellular immunity to viral infection is that CD8$^+$ CTL memory is long-lived and does not wane in an environment that contains no detectable priming antigen. This result suggests that memory, at least in the viral system we have studied, is due to the generation of antigen-independent memory T cells. This does not mean that slight or recurrent antigen is bad. Certainly re-exposure will increase the frequency of specific CTLp. However, the point should be made that, at least for the CD8$^+$ T cell compartment, the presence of the original priming antigen is not absolutely essential to maintain memory cells. This is an important concept not only for a fuller understanding of immunological memory, but also for the development of effective vaccination strategies.

References

1. Ahmed, R. (1992). Immunological memory against viruses. *Semin. Immunol.* 4: 105–109.
2. Ahmed, R., A. Salmi, L. D. Butler, J. M. Chiller, and M. B. A. Oldstone. (1984). Selection of genetic variants of lymphocytic choriomeningitis virus in spleens of persistently infected mice. Role in suppression of cytotoxic T lymphocyte response and viral persistence. *J. Exp. Med.* 160: 521–540.
3. Beverley, P. C. L. (1990). Human T cell memory. *Curr. Top. Microbiol. Immunol.* 159: 111–122.
4. Bradley, L. M., M. Croft, and S. L. Swain. (1993). T cell memory: new perspectives. *Immunol. Today.* 14: 197–199.
5. Budd, R. C., J. C. Cerottini, C. Horvath, C. Bron, T. Pedrazzini, R. C. Howe, and H. R. MacDonald. (1987). Distribution of virgin and memory T lymphocytes. Stable acquisition of the Pgp-1 glycoprotein concomitant with antigenic stimulation. *J. Immunol.* 138: 3120–3129.
6. Celada, F. (1971). The cellular basis of immunologic memory. *Prog. Allergy.* 15: 223–267.
7. Cerottini, J. C. and H. R. MacDonald. (1989). The cellular basis of T cell memory. *Ann. Rev. Immunol.* 7: 77–89.
8. Culty, M. K., K. Miyake, P. W. Kincade, E. Silorski, E. C. Butcher, and C. B. Underhill. (1990). The hyaluronate receptor is a member of the CD44 (H-CAM) family of cell surface glycoproteins. *J.Cell Biol.* 111: 2765–2774.

9. Feldbush, T. L. (1973). Antigen modulation of the immune response. The decline of immunological memory in the absence of continuing antigenic stimulation. *Cell. Immunol.* 8: 435–444.

10. Gray, D. and P. Matzinger. (1992). T cell memory is short-lived in the absence of antigen. *J. Exp. Med.* 174: 969–974.

11. Gray, D. and H. Skarvall. (1988). B cell memory is short-lived in the absence of antigen. *Nature.* 336: 707–2.

12. Haynes, B. F., M. J. Telen, L. P. Hale, and S. M. Denning. (1989). CD44—a molecule involved in leukocyte adherence and T cell activation. *Immunol. Today* 10: 423–428.

13. Jamieson, B. D. and R. Ahmed. (1989). T cell memory: long-term persistence of virus-specific cytotoxic T cells. *J. Exp. Med.* 169: 1993–2005.

14. Klaus, G. G. B., J. H. Humphrey, A. Kunkl, and D. W. Dongworth. (1980). The follicular dendritic cell: its role in antigen presentation in the generation of immunological memory. *Immunol. Rev.* 53: 1–28.

15. Lau, L. L., B. D. Jamieson, T. Somasundaram, and R. Ahmed. (1994). Cytotoxic T cell memory without antigen. *Nature.* 369: 648–652.

16. MacDonald, H. R., R. C. Budd, and J. C. Cerottini. (1990). Pgp-1 (Ly-24) as a marker of murine memory T lymphocytes. *Curr. Top. Microbiol. Immunol.* 159: 97–109.

17. Mackay, C. R. (1992). Migration pathways and immunologic memory among T lymphocytes. *Semin. Immunol.* 4:51–58.

18. Matloubian, M., S. R. Kolhekar, T. Somasundaram, and R. Ahmed. (1993). Molecular determinants of macrophage tropism and viral persistence: importance of single amino acid changes in the polymerase and glycoprotein of lymphocytic choriomeningitis virus. *J. Virol.* 67: 7340–7349.

19. Matloubian, M., S. R. Kolhekar, T. Somasundaram, and R. Ahmed. (1993). Molecular determinants of macrophage tropism and viral persistence: importance of single amino acid changes in the polymerase and glycoprotein of lymphocytic choriomeningitis virus. *J. Virol.* 67: 7340–7349.

20. Matloubian, M., T. Somasundaram, S. R. Kohekar, R. Selvakuman, and R. Ahmed. (1990). Genetic basis of viral persistence: single amino acid change in the viral glycoprotein affects ability of lymphocytic choriomeningitis virus to persist in adult mice. *J. Exp. Med.* 172: 1043–1048.

21. Miyake, K., C. B. Underhill, J. Lesley, and P. W. Kincade. (1990). Hyaluronate can function as a cell adhesion molecule and CD44 participates in hyaluronate recognition. *J. Exp. Med.* 172: 69–75.

22. Oehen, S., H. Waldner, M. Kundig, H. Hengartner, and R. M. Zinkernagel. (1992). Antivirally protective cytotoxic T cell memory to lymphocytic choriomeningitis virus is governed by persisting antigen. *J. Exp. Med.* 176: 1273–1281.

23. Sprent, J. H. Lifespans of naive, effector, and memory lymphocytes. (1993). *Curr. Opin. Immunol.* 5: 433–438.

24. Springer, T. A. (1990). Adhesion receptors of the immune system. *Nature.* 346: 425–434.

25. Stout, R.D. and J. Suttles. (1992). T cells bearing the CD44^{hi} "memory" phenotype display characteristics of activated cells in G1 stage of the cell cycle. *Cell. Immunol.* 141: 433–443.

26. Tabi, Z., F. Lynch, R. Ceredig, R. Allan, and P. C. Doherty. (1988). Virus-specific memory T cells are Pgp-1⁺ and can be selectively activated with phorbol ester and calcium ionophore. *Cell. Immunol.* 113: 268–277.

27. Tew, J. G., R. P. Phipps, and T. E. Mandel. (1980). The maintenance and regulation of the humoral immune response: persisting antigen and the role of follicular antigen-binding dendritic cells as accessor cells. *Immunol. Rev.* 53: 175–201.

28. Whitton, J. L., P. J. Southern, and M. B. A. Oldstone. (1988). Analyses of the cytotoxic T lymphocyte response to glycoprotein and nucleoprotein components of lymphocytic choriomeningitis virus. *Virology.* 162: 321–327.

29. Yednock, T. A. and S. D. Rosen. (1989). Lymphocyte homing. *Adv. Immunol.* 44: 313–378.

30. Zinkernagel, R.M. (1993). Immunity to viruses. pp. 1211–1250. In: Paul, W. (ed.) *Fundamental Immunology.* Raven Press, NY, Third edition.

31. Zinkernagel, R. M. (1990). Anti-viral T cell memory? *Curr. Top. Microbiol. Immunol.* 159: 65–77.

INDEX